Optimization in Medicine

Springer Series in Optimization and Its Applications

VOLUME 12

Managing Editor
Panos M. Pardalos (University of Florida)

Editor—Combinatorial Optimization
Ding-Zhu Du (University of Texas at Dallas)

Advisory Board
J. Birge (University of Chicago)
C.A. Floudas (Princeton University)
F. Giannessi (University of Pisa)
H.D. Sherali (Virginia Polytechnic and State University)
T. Terlaky (McMaster University)
Y. Ye (Stanford University)

Aims and Scope

Optimization has been expanding in all directions at an astonishing rate during the last few decades. New algorithmic and theoretical techniques have been developed, the diffusion into other disciplines has proceeded at a rapid pace, and our knowledge of all aspects of the field has grown even more profound. At the same time, one of the most striking trends in optimization is the constantly increasing emphasis on the interdisciplinary nature of the field. Optimization has been a basic tool in all areas of applied mathematics, engineering, medicine, economics and other sciences.

The *Springer Series in Optimization and Its Applications* publishes undergraduate and graduate textbooks, monographs and state-of-the-art expository works that focus on algorithms for solving optimization problems and also study applications involving such problems. Some of the topics covered include nonlinear optimization (convex and nonconvex), network flow problems, stochastic optimization, optimal control, discrete optimization, multi-objective programming, description of software packages, approximation techniques and heuristic approaches.

Carlos J. S. Alves
Panos M. Pardalos
Luis Nunes Vicente
Editors

Optimization in Medicine

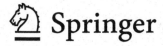 Springer

Editors

Carlos J. S. Alves
Instituto Superior Técnico
Av. Rovisco Pais 1
1049-001 Lisboa
Portugal

Panos M. Pardalos
Department of Industrial and Systems
  Engineering
University of Florida
303 Weil Hall
Gainesville, FL 32611
USA

Luis Nunes Vicente
Departamento de Matemática
Faculdade de Ciências e Tecnologia
Universidade de Coimbra
3001-454 Coimbra
Portugal

Managing Editor:

Panos M. Pardalos
University of Florida

Editor/Combinatorial Optimization

Ding-Zhu Du
University of Texas at Dallas

ISBN 978-1-4419-2517-6   e-ISBN 978-0-387-73299-2
DOI:10.1007/978-0-387-73299-2

Mathematics Subject Classification (2000): 49XX, 46N60

Printed on acid-free paper.

9 8 7 6 5 4 3 2 1

springer.com

Preface

Optimization has become pervasive in medicine. The application of computing to medical applications has opened many challenging issues and problems for both the medical computing field and the mathematical community. Mathematical techniques (continuous and discrete) are playing a key role with increasing importance in understanding several fundamental problems in medicine. Naturally, optimization is a fundamentally important tool due to the limitation of the resources involved and the need for better decision making.

The book starts with two papers on Intensity Modulated Radiation Therapy (IMRT). The first paper, by R. Acosta, M. Ehrgott, A. Holder, D. Nevin, J. Reese, and B. Salter, discusses an important subproblem in the design of radiation plans, the selection of beam directions. The manuscript compares different heuristic methods for beam selection on a clinical case and studies the effect of various dose calculation grid resolutions. The next paper, by M. Ehrgott, H. W. Hamacher, and M. Nußbaum, reviews several contributions on the decomposition of matrices as a model for rearranging leaves on a multileaf collimator. Such a process is essential for block radiation in IMRT in order to achieve desirable intensity profiles. Additionally, they present a new approach for minimizing the number of decomposition segments by sequentially solving this problem in polynomial time with respect to fixed decomposition times.

The book continues with a paper by G. Deng and M. Ferris on the formulation of the day-to-day radiation therapy treatment planning problem as a dynamic program. The authors consider errors due to variations in the positioning of the patient and apply neuro-dynamic programming to compute approximate solutions for the dynamic optimization problems. The fourth paper, by H. Fohlin, L. Kliemann, and A. Srivastav, considers the seed reconstruction problem in brachytherapy as a minimum-weight perfect matching problem in a hypergraph. The problem is modeled as an integer linear program for which the authors develop an algorithm based on a randomized rounding scheme and a greedy approach.

The book also covers other types of medical applications. For instance, in the paper by S. Sabesan, N. Chakravarthy, L. Good, K. Tsakalis, P. Pardalos, and L. Iasemidis, the authors propose an application of global optimization in the selection of critical brain sites prior to an epileptic seizure. The paper shows the advantages of using optimization (in particular nonconvex quadratic programming) in combination with measures of EEG dynamics, such as Lyapunov exponents, phase and energy, for long-term prediction of epileptic seizures.

E. K. Lee presents the optimization-classification models within discriminant analysis, to develop predictive rules for large heterogeneous biological and medical data sets. As mentioned by the author, classification models are critical to medical advances as they can be used in genomic, cell molecular, and system level analysis to assist in early prediction, diagnosis and detection of diseases, as well as for intervention and monitoring. A wide range of applications are described in the paper.

This book also includes two papers on inverse problems with applications to medical imaging. The paper by A. K. Louis presents an overview of several techniques that lead to robust algorithms for imaging reconstruction from the measured data. In particular, the inversion of the Radon transform is considered as a model case of inversion. In this paper, a reconstruction of the inside of a *surprise egg* is presented as a numerical example for 3D X-Ray reconstruction from real data. In the paper by M. Malinen, T. Huttunen, and J. Kaipio, an inverse problem related to ultrasound surgery is considered in an optimization framework that aims to control the optimal thermal dose to apply, for instance, in the treatment of breast cancer. Two alternative procedures (a scanning path optimization algorithm and a feedforward-feedback control method) are discussed in detail with numerical examples in 2D and 3D.

We would like to thank the authors for their contributions. It would not have been possible to reach the quality of this publication without the contributions of the many anonymous referees involved in the revision and acceptance process of the submitted manuscripts. Our gratitude is extended to them as well.

This book was generated mostly from invited talks given at the Workshop on Optimization in Medicine, July 20-22, 2005, which took place at the Institute of Biomedical Research in Light and Image (IBILI), University of Coimbra, Portugal. The workshop was organized under the auspices of the International Center for Mathematics (CIM, http://www.cim.pt) as part of the 2005 CIM Thematic Term on Optimization.

Finally, we would like to thank Ana Luísa Custódio (FCT/UNL) for her help in the organization of the workshop and Pedro C. Martins (ISCAC/IPC) and João M. M. Patrício (ESTT/IPT) for their invaluable editorial support.

Coimbra,   *C. J. S. Alves*
May 2007   *P. M. Pardalos*
                                                                 L. N. Vicente

Contents

List of Contributors

Ryan Acosta
Institute for Computational and
Mathematical Engineering,
Stanford University
Stanford, California, USA.
raacosta@stanford.edu

Niranjan Chakravarthy
Department of Electrical Engineer-
ing, Fulton School of Engineering,
Arizona State University,
Tempe, AZ 85281, USA.
niranjan.chakravarthy@asu.edu

Geng Deng
Department of Mathematics,
University of Wisconsin at Madison,
480 Lincoln Dr., Madison, WI 53706,
USA.
geng@cs.wisc.edu

Matthias Ehrgott
Department of Engineering Science,
The University of Auckland,
Auckland, New Zealand.
m.ehrgott@auckland.ac.nz

Michael C. Ferris
Computer Sciences Department,
University of Wisconsin at Madison,
1210 W. Dayton Street,
Madison, WI 53706, USA.
ferris@cs.wisc.edu

Helena Fohlin
Department of Oncology, Linköping
University Hospital,
581 85 Linköping, Sweden.
helena.fohlin@lio.se

Levi Good
The Harrington Department of
Bioengineering, Fulton School of
Engineering, Arizona State
University, Tempe, AZ 85281, USA.
levi.good@asu.edu

Horst W. Hamacher
Fachbereich Mathematik, Technische
Universität Kaiserslautern,
Kaiserslautern, Germany.
hamacher@mathematik.uni-kl.de

Allen Holder
Department of Mathematics, Trinity
University, and
Department of Radiation Oncology,
University of Texas Health
Science Center, San Antonio, Texas,
USA.
aholder@trinity.edu

Tomi Huttunen
Department of Physics, University of
Kuopio, P.O. Box 1627,
FIN-70211, Finland.

Leon Iasemidis
The Harrington Department of
Bioengineering, Fulton School of
Engineering, Arizona State
University, Tempe, AZ 85281, USA.
leon.iasemidis@asu.edu

Jari P. Kaipio
Department of Physics, University of
Kuopio, P.O. Box 1627,
FIN-70211, Finland.

Lasse Kliemann
Institut für Informatik, Christian–
Albrechts–Universität zu Kiel,
Christian-Albrechts-Platz 4,
D–24098 Kiel, Germany.
lki@numerik.uni-kiel.de

Eva K. Lee
Center for Operations Research in
Medicine and HealthCare,
School of Industrial and
Systems Engineering,
Georgia Institute of Technology,
Atlanta, GA 30332-0205, USA.
eva.lee@isye.gatech.edu

Alfred K. Louis
Department of Mathematics,
Saarland University,
66041 Saarbrücken, Germany.
louis@num.uni-sb.de

Matti Malinen
Department of Physics, University of
Kuopio, P.O. Box 1627,
FIN-70211, Finland.
Matti.Malinen@uku.fi

Daniel Nevin
Department of Computer Science,
Texas A&M University,
College Station, Texas, USA.
dnevin@tamu.edu

Marc Nußbaum
Fachbereich Mathematik, Technische
Universität Kaiserslautern,
Kaiserslautern, Germany.

Panos M. Pardalos
Department of Industrial and
Systems Engineering,
University of Florida, Gainesville,
FL 32611, USA.
pardalos@ufl.edu

Josh Reese
Department of Mathematics,
Trinity University,
San Antonio, Texas, USA.
jreese@trinity.edu

Shivkumar Sabesan
Department of Electrical Engineer-
ing, Fulton School of Engineering,
Arizona State University,
Tempe, AZ 85281, USA.
shivkumar.sabesan@asu.edu

Bill Salter
Department of Radiation Oncology,
University of Utah Huntsman
Cancer Institute,
Salt Lake City, Utah, USA.
bill.salter@hci.utah.edu

Anand Srivastav
Institut für Informatik, Christian–
Albrechts–Universität zu Kiel,
Christian-Albrechts-Platz 4,
D–24098 Kiel, Germany.
asr@numerik.uni-kiel.de

Kostas Tsakalis
Department of Electrical Engineer-
ing, Fulton School of Engineering,
Arizona State University, Tempe,
AZ 85281, USA.
tsakalis@asu.edu

The influence of dose grid resolution on beam selection strategies in radiotherapy treatment design

Ryan Acosta[1], Matthias Ehrgott[2], Allen Holder[3], Daniel Nevin[4], Josh Reese[5], and Bill Salter[6]

[1] Institute for Computational and Mathematical Engineering, Stanford University, Stanford, California, USA. `raacosta@stanford.edu`.
[2] Department of Engineering Science, The University of Auckland, Auckland, New Zealand. `m.ehrgott@auckland.ac.nz`.
[3] Department of Mathematics, Trinity University, and Department of Radiation Oncology, University of Texas Health Science Center, San Antonio, Texas, USA. `aholder@trinity.edu`.
[4] Department of Computer Science, Texas A&M University, College Station, Texas, USA. `dnevin@tamu.edu`.
[5] Department of Mathematics, Trinity University, San Antonio, Texas, USA. `jreese@trinity.edu`.
[6] Department of Radiation Oncology, University of Utah Huntsman Cancer Institute, Salt Lake City, Utah, USA. `bill.salter@hci.utah.edu`.

Summary. The design of a radiotherapy treatment includes the selection of beam angles (geometry problem), the computation of a fluence pattern for each selected beam angle (intensity problem), and finding a sequence of configurations of a multileaf collimator to deliver the treatment (realization problem). While many mathematical optimization models and algorithms have been proposed for the intensity problem and (to a lesser extent) the realization problem, this is not the case for the geometry problem. In clinical practice, beam directions are manually selected by a clinician and are typically based on the clinician's experience. Solving the beam selection problem optimally is beyond the capability of current optimization algorithms and software. However, heuristic methods have been proposed. In this paper we study the influence of dose grid resolution on the performance of these heuristics for a clinical case. Dose grid resolution refers to the spatial arrangement and size of dose calculation voxels. In particular, we compare the solutions obtained by the heuristics with those achieved by a clinician using a commercial planning system. Our results show that dose grid resolution has a considerable influence on the performance of most heuristics.

Keywords: Intensity modulated radiation therapy, beam angle selection, heuristics, vector quantization, dose grid resolution, medical physics, optimization.

1 Introduction

Radiotherapy is the treatment of cancerous and displasiac tissues with ionizing radiation that can damage the DNA of cells. While non-cancerous cells are able to repair slightly damaged DNA, the heightened state of reproduction that cancerous cells are in means that small amounts of DNA damage can render them incapable of reproducing. The goal of radiotherapy is to exploit this therapeutic advantage by focusing the radiation so that enough dose is delivered to the targeted region to kill the cancerous cells while surrounding anatomical structures are spared and maintained at minimal damage levels.

In the past, it was reasonable for a clinician to design radiotherapy treatments manually due to the limited capabilities of radiotherapy equipment. However, with the advent of intensity modulated radiotherapy (IMRT), the number of possible treatment options and the number of parameters have become so immense that they exceed the capabilities of even the most experienced treatment planner. Therefore, optimization methods and computer assisted planning tools have become a necessity. IMRT treatments use multileaf collimators to shape the beam and control, or modulate the dose that is delivered along a fixed direction of focus. IMRT allows beams to be decomposed into a (large) number of sub-beams, for which the intensity can be chosen individually. In addition, movement of the treatment couch and gantry allows radiation to be focused from almost any location on a (virtual) sphere around the target volume. For background on radiotherapy and IMRT we refer to [24] and [29].

Designing an optimal treatment means deciding on a huge number of parameters. The design process is therefore usually divided into three phases, namely 1) the selection of directions from which to focus radiation on the patient, 2) the selection of fluence patterns (amount of radiation delivered) for the directions selected in phase one, and 3) the selection of a mechanical delivery sequence that efficiently administers the treatment. Today there are many optimization methods for the intensity problem, with suggested models including linear (e.g., [21, 23]), integer (e.g., [13, 19]), and nonlinear (e.g., [15, 27]) formulations as well as models of multiobjective optimization (e.g., [7, 9, 22]).

Similarly, algorithms have been proposed to find good multileaf collimator sequences to reduce treatment times and minimize between-leaf leakage and background dose [3, 25, 31]. Such algorithms are in use in existing radiotherapy equipment. Moreover, researchers have studied the mathematical structure of these problems to improve algorithm design or to establish the optimality of an algorithm [1, 2, 11].

In this paper we consider the geometry problem. The literature on this topic reveals a different picture than that of the intensity and realization problems. While a number of methods were proposed, there was a lack of understanding of the underlying mathematics. The authors in [4] propose a mathematical framework that unifies the approaches found in the literature.

The focus of this paper is how different approximations of the anatomical dose affect beam selection.

The beam selection problem is important for several reasons. First, changing beam directions during treatment is time consuming, and the number of directions is typically limited to reduce the overall treatment time. Since most clinics treat patients steadily throughout the day, patients are usually treated in daily sessions of 15-30 minutes to make sure that demand is satisfied. Moreover, short treatments are desirable because lengthy procedures increase the likelihood of a patient altering his or her position on the couch, which can lead to inaccurate and potentially dangerous treatments. Lastly, and perhaps most importantly, beam directions must be judiciously selected so as to minimize the radiation exposure to life-critical tissues and organs, while maximizing the dose to the targeted tumor.

Selecting the beam directions is currently done manually, and it typically requires several trial-and-error iterations between selecting beam directions and calculating fluence patterns until a satisfactory treatment is designed. Hence, the process is time intensive and subject to the experience of the clinician. Finding a suitable collection of directions can take as much as several hours. The goal of using an optimization method to identify quality directions is to remove the dependency on a clinician's experience and to alleviate the tedious repetitive process of selecting angles.

To evaluate the dose distribution in the patient, it is necessary to calculate how radiation is deposited into the patient. There are numerous dose models in the literature, with the gold standard being a Monte Carlo technique that simulates each particle's path through the anatomy. We use an accurate 3D dose model developed in [18] and [17]. This so-called finite sized pencil beam approach is currently in clinical use in numerous commercial planning systems in radiation treatment clinics throughout the world.

Positions within the anatomy where dose is calculated may be referred to as *dose points*. Because each patient image represents a slice of the anatomy of varying thickness, and hence, each dose point represents a 3D hyper-rectangle whose dimensions are decided by both the slice thickness and the spacing of the dose points within a slice, such dose calculation points are also referred to as *voxels* in recognition of their 3D, or volumetric, nature. We point out that the terms dose point and dose voxel are used interchangeably throughout this text.

The authors in [16] study the effects of different dose (constraint) point placement algorithms on the optimized treatment planning solution (for given beam directions) using open and wedged beams. They find very different dose patterns and conclude that 2000-9000 points are needed for 10 to 30 CT slices in order to obtain good results. The goal of this paper is to evaluate the influence of dose voxel spacing on automated beam selection.

In Section 2 we introduce the beam selection problem, state some of its properties and define the underlying fluence map optimization problem used in this study. In Section 3 we summarize the beam selection methods considered in the numerical experiments. These are set covering and scoring methods as well as a vector quantization technique. Section 4 contains the numerical results and Section 5 briefly summarizes the achievements.

2 The beam selection problem

First we note that throughout this paper the terms beam, direction, and angle are used interchangeably. The beam selection problem is to find N positions for the patient and gantry from which the treatment will be delivered. The gantry of a linear accelerator can rotate around the patient in a great circle and the couch can rotate in the plane of its surface. There are physical restrictions on the directions that can be used because some couch and gantry positions result in collisions.

In this paper we consider co-planar treatments. That is, beam angles are chosen on a great circle around the CT-slice of the body that contains the center of the tumor. We let $\mathcal{A} = \{a_j : j \in J\}$ be a candidate collection of angles from which we will select N to treat the patient, where we typically consider $\mathcal{A} = \{i\pi/36 : i = 0, 1, 2, \dots, 71\}$. To evaluate a collection of angles, a judgment function is needed that describes how well a patient can be treated with that collection of angles [4].

We denote the power set of $\mathcal{A}$ by $\mathcal{P}(\mathcal{A})$ and the nonnegative extended reals by $\mathbb{R}_+^*$. A *judgment function* is a function $f : \mathcal{P}(\mathcal{A}) \to \mathbb{R}_+^*$ with the property that $\mathcal{A}' \supseteq \mathcal{A}''$ implies $f(\mathcal{A}') \leq f(\mathcal{A}'')$. The value of $f(\mathcal{A}')$ is the optimal value of an optimization problem that decides a fluence pattern for angles $\mathcal{A}'$, i.e., for any $\mathcal{A}' \in \mathcal{P}(\mathcal{A})$,

$$f(\mathcal{A}') = \min\{z(x) : x \in X(\mathcal{A}')\}, \tag{1}$$

where z maps a fluence pattern $x \in X(\mathcal{A}')$, the set of feasible fluence patterns for angles $\mathcal{A}'$, into $\mathbb{R}_+^*$. As pointed out above, there is a large amount of literature on modeling and calculating f, i.e., solving the intensity problem. In fact, all commercial planning systems use an optimization routine to decide a fluence pattern, but the model and calculation method differ from system to system [30].

We assume that if a feasible treatment cannot be achieved with a given set of angles $\mathcal{A}'$ ($X(\mathcal{A}') = \emptyset$) then $f(\mathcal{A}') = \infty$. We further assume that x is a vector in $\mathbb{R}^{|\mathcal{A}| \times I}$, where I is the number of sub-beams of a beam, and make the tacit assumptions that $x_{(a,i)} = 0$ for all sub-beams i of any angle $a \in \mathcal{A} \setminus \mathcal{A}'$. The non-decreasing behavior of f with respect to set inclusion is then modeled via the set of feasible fluence patterns $X(\mathcal{A})$ by assuming that $X(\mathcal{A}'') \subseteq X(\mathcal{A}')$ whenever $\mathcal{A}'' \subseteq \mathcal{A}'$. We say that the fluence pattern x is optimal for $\mathcal{A}'$ if $f(\mathcal{A}') = z(x)$ and $x \in X(\mathcal{A}')$. All fluence map optimization models share the property that the quality of a treatment cannot deteriorate if more angles are used. The result that a judgment function is non-decreasing with respect to the number of angles follows from the definition of a judgment function and the above assumptions, see [4].

A judgment function is defined by the data that forms the optimization problem in (1). This data includes a dose operator D, a prescription P, and an objective function z. We let $d_{(k,a,i)}$ be the rate at which radiation along sub-beam i in angle a is deposited into dose point k, and we assume that $d_{(k,a,i)}$ is nonnegative for each (k,a,i). These rates are patient-specific constants and the operator that maps a fluence pattern into anatomical dose (measured in Grays, Gy) is linear. We let D be the matrix whose elements are $d_{(k,a,i)}$, where the rows are indexed by k and the columns by (a,i). The linear operator $x \mapsto Dx$ maps the fluence pattern x to the dose that is deposited into the patient (see, e.g., [12] for a justification of the linearity). To avoid unnecessary notation we use $\sum_i$ to indicate that we are summing over the sub-beams in an angle. So, $\sum_i x_{(a,i)}$ is the total exposure (or fluence) for angle a, and $\sum_i d_{(k,a,i)}$ is the aggregated rate at which dose is deposited into dose point k from angle a.

There are a variety of forms that a prescription can have, each dependent on what the optimization problem is attempting to accomplish. Since the purpose of this paper is to compare the effect of dose point resolution on various approaches to the beam selection problem, we focus on one particular judgment function. Let us partition the set of dose voxels into those that are being targeted for dose deposition (i.e., within a tumor), those that are within a critical structure (i.e., very sensitive locations, such as brainstem, identified for dose avoidance), and those that represent normal tissue (i.e., non-specific healthy tissues which should be avoided, but are not as sensitive or important as critical structures). We denote the set of targeted dose voxels by T, the collection of dose points in the critical regions by C, and the remaining dose points by N. We further let D_T, D_C, and D_N be the submatrices of D such that $D_T x$, $D_C x$, and $D_N x$ map the fluence pattern x into the targeted region, the critical structures, and the normal tissue, respectively. The prescription consists of TLB and TUB, which are vectors of lower and upper bounds on the targeted dose points, CUB, which is a vector of upper bounds on the critical structures, and NUB, which is a vector of upper bounds on the normal tissue. The judgment function is defined by the following linear program [8].

$$
\left.
\begin{aligned}
f(\mathcal{A}') = \min \omega\alpha + \beta + \gamma \\
TLB - e\alpha \le D_T x \\
D_T x \le TUB \\
D_C x \le CUB + e\beta \\
D_N x \le NUB + e\gamma \\
TLB \ge e\alpha \\
-CUB \le e\beta \\
x, \gamma \ge 0 \\
\sum_i x_{(a,i)} = 0 \text{ for all } a \in \mathcal{A}\backslash\mathcal{A}'.
\end{aligned}
\right\}
\tag{2}
$$

Here e is the vector of ones of appropriate dimension. The scalars α, β, and γ measure the worst deviation from TLB, CUB, and NUB for any single dose voxel in the target, the critical structures, and the normal tissue, respectively. For a fixed judgment function such as (2), the N-beam selection problem is

$$\min\{f(\mathcal{A}') - f(\mathcal{A}) : \mathcal{A}' \in \mathcal{P}(\mathcal{A}), |\mathcal{A}'| = N\}$$
$$= \min\{f(\mathcal{A}') : \mathcal{A}' \in \mathcal{P}(\mathcal{A}), |\mathcal{A}'| = N\} - f(\mathcal{A}). \qquad (3)$$

Note that the beam selection problem is the minimization of a judgment function f. The value of the judgment function itself is the optimal value of an optimization problem such as (2) that in turn has an objective function $z(x)$ to be minimized.

The minimization problem (3) can be stated as an extension of the optimization problem that defines f using binary variables. Let

$$y_a = \begin{cases} 1 \text{ angle } a \text{ is selected,} \\ 0 \text{ otherwise.} \end{cases}$$

Then the beam selection problem becomes

$$\left.\begin{array}{c} \min z(x) \\ \sum_{a \in \mathcal{A}} y_a = N \\ \sum_i x_{(i,a)} \le My_a \text{ for all } a \in \mathcal{A} \\ x \in X(\mathcal{A}), \end{array}\right\} \qquad (4)$$

where M is a sufficiently large constant.

While (4) is a general model that combines the optimal selection of beams with the optimization of their fluence patterns, such problems are currently intractable because they are beyond modern solution capabilities. Note that there are between 1.4×10^7 and 5.4×10^{11} subsets of $\{i\pi/36 : i = 0, 1, 2, \ldots, 71\}$ for clinically relevant values of N ranging from 5 to 10. In any study where the solution of these MIPs is attempted [5, 13, 14, 19, 28], the set $|\mathcal{A}|$ is severely restricted so that the number of binary variables is manageable. This fact has led researchers to investigate heuristics.

In the following section we present the heuristics that we include in our computational results in the framework of beam selectors introduced in [4]. The function $g : \mathcal{W} \to \mathcal{V}$ is a *beam selector* if $\mathcal{W}$ and $\mathcal{V}$ are subsets of $\mathcal{P}(\mathcal{A})$ and $g(W) \subseteq W$ for all $W \in \mathcal{W}$. A beam selector $g : \mathcal{W} \to \mathcal{V}$ maps every collection of angles in $\mathcal{W}$ to a subcollection of *selected angles*. An *N-beam selector* is a beam selector with $|\cup_{W \in \mathcal{W}} g(W)| = N$. A beam selector is *informed* if it is defined in terms of the value of a judgment function and it is *weakly informed* if it is defined in terms of the data (D, P, z). A beam selector is otherwise *uninformed*. If g is defined in terms of a random variable, then g is *stochastic*.

An important observation is that for any collection of angles $\mathcal{A}' \subset \mathcal{A}$ there is not necessarily a unique optimal fluence pattern, which means that informed beam selectors are solver dependent. An example in Section 5 of [4] shows how radically different optimal fluence patterns obtained by different solvers for the same judgment function can be.

There are several heuristic beam selection techniques in the literature. Each heuristic approach to the problem can be interpreted as choosing a best beam selector of a specified type as described in [4]. Additional references on methods not used in this study and methods for which the original papers do not provide sufficient detail to reproduce their results can be found in [4].

3 The beam selection methods

We first present the set covering approach developed by [5]. An angle a covers the dose point k if $\sum_i d_{(k,a,i)} \geq \varepsilon$. For each $k \in T$, let $\mathcal{A}_k^\varepsilon = \{a \in \mathcal{A} : a \text{ cover dose point } k\}$. A (set-covering) SC-$N$-beam selector is an N-beam selector having the form

$$g_{sc} : \{\mathcal{A}_k^\varepsilon : k \in T\} \to \bigcup_{k \in T} (\mathcal{P}(\mathcal{A}_k^\varepsilon) \backslash \emptyset).$$

Two observations are important:

1. We have $\mathcal{A}_k^\varepsilon = \mathcal{A}$ for all $k \in T$ if and only if $0 \leq \varepsilon \leq \varepsilon^* := \min\{\sum_i d_{(k,a,i)} : k \in T, a \in \mathcal{A}\}$. The most common scenario is that each targeted dose point is covered by every angle.
2. Since g_{sc} cannot map to $\emptyset$, the mapping has to select at least one angle to cover each targeted dose point.

It was shown in [4] that for $0 \leq \varepsilon \leq \varepsilon^*$, the set covering approach to beam selection is equivalent to the beam selection problem (3). This equivalence means that we cannot solve the set-covering beam selection problem efficiently. However, heuristically it is possible to restrict the optimization to subsets of SC-N-beam selectors. This was done in [5]. The second observation allows the formulation of a traditional set covering problem to identify a single g_{sc}. For each targeted dose point k, let $q_{(k,a,i)}$ be 1 if sub-beam i in angle a covers dose point k, and 0 otherwise. For each angle a, define

$$c_a = \begin{cases} \sum_{k \in C} \sum_i \frac{q_{(k,a,i)}}{CUB_k} & \text{if } C \neq \emptyset, \\ 0 & \text{if } C = \emptyset, \end{cases} \tag{5}$$

and

$$\hat{c}_a = \begin{cases} \sum_{k \in C} \sum_i \frac{q_{(k,a,i)} \cdot d_{(k,a,i)}}{CUB_k} & \text{if } C \neq \emptyset, \\ 0 & \text{if } C = \emptyset, \end{cases} \tag{6}$$

where CUB is part of the prescription in (2). The costs c_a and $\hat{c}_a$ are large if sub-beams of a intersect a critical structure that has a small upper bound.

Cost coefficients $\hat{c}_a$ are additionally scaled by the rate at which the dose is deposited into dose point k from sub-beam (a, i).

The associated set covering problems are

$$\min \left\{ \sum_a c_a y_a : \sum_a q_{(k,a)} y_a \geq 1, \ k \in T, \ \sum_a y_a = N, \ y_a \in \{0, 1\} \right\} \quad (7)$$

and

$$\min \left\{ \sum_a \hat{c}_a y_a : \sum_a q_{(k,a)} y_a \geq 1, \ k \in T, \ \sum_a y_a = N, \ y_a \in \{0, 1\} \right\}. \quad (8)$$

The angles for which $y_a^* = 1$ in an optimal solution y^* of (7) or (8) are selected and define a particular SC-N-beam selector. Note that such N-beam selectors are weakly informed, if not at all informed, as they use the data but do not evaluate f.

These particular set covering problems are generally easy to solve. In fact, in the common situation of $\mathcal{A}_k^\varepsilon = \mathcal{A}$ for $k \in T$, (7) and (8) reduce to selecting N angles in order of increasing c_a or $\hat{c}_a$, respectively. This leads us to scoring techniques for the beam selection problem.

We can interpret c_a or $\hat{c}_a$ as a score of angle a. A (scoring) S-N-beam selector is an N-beam selector $g_s : \{\mathcal{A}\} \to \mathcal{P}(\mathcal{A})$. It is not surprising that the scoring approach is equivalent to the beam selection problem. The difficulty here lies in defining scores that accurately predict angles that are used in an optimal treatment.

The first scoring approach we consider is found in [20], where each angle is assigned the score

$$c_a = \frac{1}{|T|} \sum_{k \in T} \sum_i \left(\frac{d_{(k,a,i)} \cdot \hat{x}_{(a,i)}}{TG} \right)^2, \quad (9)$$

where

$$\hat{x}_{(a,i)} = \min\{\min\{CUB_k/d_{(k,a,i)} : k \in C\}, \ \min\{NUB_k/d_{(k,a,i)} : k \in N\}\}$$

and TG is a goal dose to the target and $TLB \leq TG \leq TUB$. An angle's score increases as the sub-beams that comprise the angle are capable of delivering more radiation to the target without violating the restrictions placed on the non-targeted region(s). Here, high scores are desirable. The scoring technique uses the bounds on the non-targeted tissues to form constraints, and the score represents how well the target can be treated while satisfying these constraints. This is the reverse of the perspective in (7) and (8). Nevertheless, mathematically, every scoring technique is a set covering problem [4].

Another scoring method is found in [26]. Letting x^* be an optimal fluence pattern for $\mathcal{A}$, the authors in [26] define the entropy of an angle by $\delta_a := -\sum_i x_{(a,i)}^* \ln x_{(a,i)}^*$ and the score of a is

$$c_a = 1 - \frac{\delta_a - \min\{\delta_a : a \in \mathcal{A}\}}{\max\{\delta_a : a \in \mathcal{A}\}}. \tag{10}$$

In this approach, an angle's score is high if the optimal fluence pattern of an angle's sub-beams is uniformly high. So, an angle with a single high-fluence sub-beam would likely have a lower score than an angle with a more uniform fluence pattern. Unlike the scoring procedure in [20], this technique is informed since it requires an evaluation of f.

The last of the techniques we consider is based on the image compression technique called vector quantization [10] (see [6] for further information on vector quantization). $\mathcal{A}'$ is a contiguous subset of $\mathcal{A}$ if $\mathcal{A}'$ is an ordered subset of the form $\{a_j, a_{j+1}, \ldots, a_{j+r}\}$. A contiguous partition of $\mathcal{A}$ is a collection of contiguous subsets of $\mathcal{A}$ that partition $\mathcal{A}$, and we let $\mathcal{W}_{vq}(N)$ be the collection of N element contiguous partitions of $\mathcal{A}$. A VQ-N-beam selector is a function of the form

$$g_{vq} : \{W_j : j = 1, 2, \ldots, N\} \rightarrow \{\{a_j\} : a_j \in W_j\},$$

where $\{W_j : j = 1, 2, \ldots, N\} \in \mathcal{W}_{vq}(N)$.

The image of W_j is a singleton $\{a_j\}$, and we usually write a_j instead of $\{a_j\}$. The VQ-N-beam selector relies on the probability that an angle is used in an optimal treatment. Letting $\alpha(a)$ be this probability, we have that the *distortion* of a quantizer is

$$\sum_{j=1}^{N} \sum_{a \in W_j} \alpha(a) \cdot \|a - g_{vq}(W_j)\|_2.$$

Once the probability distribution α is known, a VQ-N-beam selector is calculated to minimize distortion. In the special case of a continuous $\mathcal{A}$, the authors in [6] show that the selected angles are the centers-of-mass of the contiguous sets. We mimic this behavior in the discrete setting by defining

$$g_{vq}(W_j) = \frac{\sum_{a \in W_j} a \cdot \alpha(a)}{\sum_{a \in W_j} \alpha(a)}. \tag{11}$$

This center-of-mass calculation is not exact for discrete sets since the center-of-mass may not be an element of the contiguous set. Therefore angles not in $\mathcal{A}$ are mapped to their nearest neighbor, with ties being mapped to the larger element of $\mathcal{A}$.

Vector quantization heuristics select a contiguous partition from which a single VQ-N-beam selector is created according to condition (11). The process in [10] starts by selecting the zero angle as the beginning of the first contiguous set. The endpoints of the contiguous sets are found by forming the cumulative density and evenly dividing its range into N intervals. To improve this, we could use the same rule and rotate the starting angle through the 72 candidates. We could then evaluate f over these sets of beams and take the smallest value.

The success of the vector quantization approach directly relies on the ability of the probability distribution to accurately gauge the likelihood of an angle being used in an optimal N-beam treatment. An immediate idea is to make a weakly informed probability distribution by normalizing the scoring techniques in (5), (6) and (9). Additionally, the scores in (10) are normalized to create an informed model of α. We test these methods in Section 4. An alternative informed probability density is suggested in [10], where the authors assume that an optimal fluence pattern x^* for $f(\mathcal{A})$ contains information about which angles should and should not be used. Let

$$\alpha(a) = \frac{\sum\limits_i x^*_{(a,i)}}{\sum\limits_{a\in\mathcal{A}}\sum\limits_i x^*_{(a,i)}}.$$

Since optimal fluence patterns are not unique, these probabilities are solver-dependent. In [4] an algorithm is given to remove this solver dependency. The algorithm transforms an optimal fluence x^* into a balanced probability density α, i.e., one that is as uniform as possible, by solving the problem

$$\text{lexmin}\,(z(x), \text{sort}(x)),\qquad(12)$$

where sort is a function that reorders the components of the vector x in a non-increasing order. The algorithm that produces the balanced solution iteratively reduces the maximum exposure time of the sub-beams that are not fixed, which intuitively means that we are re-distributing fluence over the remaining sub-beams. As the maximum fluence decreases, the fluences for some angles need to increase to guarantee an optimal treatment. The algorithm terminates as soon as the variables that are fixed by this "equalizing" process attain one of the bounds that describe an optimal treatment. At the algorithm's termination, a further reduction of sub-beam fluences whose α value is high will no longer allow an optimal treatment.

4 Numerical comparisons

In this section we numerically compare how the resolution of the dose points affects set cover (SC), scoring (S), and vector quantization (VQ) 9-beam selectors. The $\mathcal{R}$adiotherapy optim$\mathcal{A}$l $\mathcal{D}$esign software ($\mathcal{RAD}$) at http://www.trinity.edu/aholder/research/oncology/rad.html was altered to accommodate the different beam selectors. This system is written in Matlab© and links to the CPLEX© solvers (CPLEX v. 6.6. was used). The code, except for commercial packages, and all figures used in this paper (and more) are available at http://lagrange.math.trinity.edu/tumath/research/reports/misc/report97.

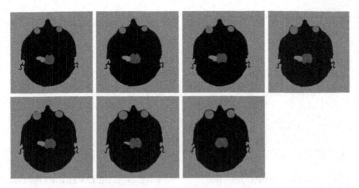

Fig. 1. The target is immediately to the left of the brainstem. The critical structures are the brain stem and the two eye sockets.

The clinical example is an acoustic neuroma in which the target is immediately adjacent to the brain stem and is desired to receive between 48.08 and 59.36 Gy. The brain stem is restricted to no more than 50 Gy and the eye sockets to less than 5 Gy. Each image represents a 1.5 mm swath of the patient, and the 7 images in Figure 1 were used, creating a 10.5 mm thickness. The full clinical set contained 110 images, but we were unable to handle the full complement because of inherent memory limitations in Matlab.

Angles are selected from $\{i\pi/36 : i = 1, 2, \ldots, 71\}$. These candidate angles were assigned twelve different values as follows. An optimal treatment (according to judgment function (2)) for the full set of candidate angles was found with CPLEX's primal, dual, and interior-point methods and a balanced solution according to (12) was also calculated. The angle values were either the average sub-beam exposure or the maximal sub-beam exposure. So, "BalancedAvg" indicates that the angle values were created from the balanced solution of a 72-angle optimal treatment, where the angle values were the average sub-beam exposure. Similar nomenclature is used for "DualMax," "PrimalAvg," and so on. This yields eight values. The scaled and unscaled set cover values in (5) and (6) were also used and are denoted by "SC1" and "SC2." The informed entropy measure in (10) is denoted by "Entropy," and the scoring technique in (9) is denoted by "S." We used $TG = 0.5(TLB + TUB)$ in (9). So, in total we tested twelve different angle values for each of the beam selectors.

The dose points were placed on 3 mm and 5 mm grids throughout the 3D patient space, and each dose point was classified by the type of tissue it represented. Since the images were spaced at 1.5 mm, we point out that dose points were not necessarily centered on the images in the superior inferior direction. The classification of whether or not a dose point was targeted, critical, or normal was accomplished by relating the dose point to the hyperrectangle in which it was contained. In a clinical setting, the anatomical dose is typically approximated by a 1 to 5 mm spacing, so the experiments are similar to clinical practice. However, as with the number of images, Matlab's

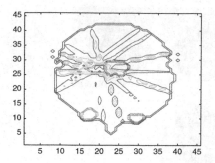

Fig. 2. The isodose contours for the balanced 72-angle treatment with 5 mm spacing.

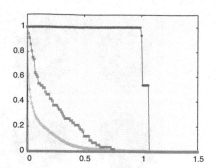

Fig. 3. The DVH for the balanced 72-angle treatment with 5 mm spacing.

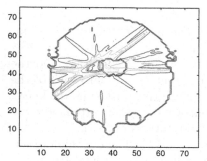

Fig. 4. The isodose contours for the balanced 72-angle treatment with 3 mm spacing.

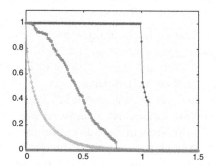

Fig. 5. The DVH for the balanced 72-angle treatment with 3 mm spacing.

memory limitation did not allow us to further increase the resolution (i.e., decrease the dose point spacing).

Treatments are judged by viewing the level curves of the radiation per slice, called *isodose curves*, and by their cumulative dose volume histogram (DVH). A dose volume histogram is a plot of percent dose (relative to TLB) versus the percent volume. The isodose curves and DVHs for the balanced 72-angle treatment are shown for the 3 mm and 5 mm resolutions in Figures 2 through 5. An ideal DVH would have the target at 100% for the entire volume and then drop immediately to zero, indicating that the target is treated exactly as specified with no under or over dosing. The curves for the critical structures would instead drop immediately to zero, meaning that they receive no radiation. The DVHs in Figures 3 and 5 follow this trend and are, therefore, clinically reasonable. The curves from upper-right to lower left are for the target, the brain stem, normal tissue, and the eye sockets. The eye socket curves drop immediately to zero as desired and appear on the axes. The 3 mm brain stem curve indicates that this structure is receiving more radiation than with the 5 mm resolution. While the fluence maps generated for

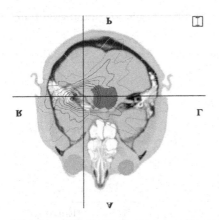

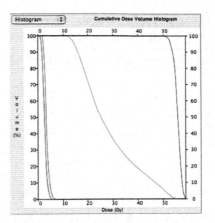

Fig. 6. The isodose contours for a clinical serial tomotherapy treatment.

Fig. 7. The DVH for a clinical serial tomotherapy treatment.

these two treatments are different, the largest part of this discrepancy is likely due to the 3 mm spacing more accurately representing the dose variation.

Figures 6 and 7 are from a commercially available, clinically used serial tomotherapy treatment system (Corvus v6.1 – Nomos Inc., Cranberry Township, PA), which uses 72 equally spaced angles (the curve for the normal tissue is not displayed). Two observations are important. First, the similarity between the DVHs of our computed solutions and Corvus' DVHs suggests that our dose model and judgment function are reasonable. Second, if our resolutions were decreased to 2 or 1.5 mm, it is likely that we would observe a brain stem curve more closely akin to that in Corvus' DVH. We point out that the judgment function and solution procedure are different for the Corvus system (and are proprietary).

A natural question is whether or not the dose point resolution affects the angle values. We expected differences, but were not clear as to how much of an effect to expect. We were intrigued to see that some of the differences were rather dramatic. The 3 mm and 5 mm "average" values are shown in Table 1.

The selected angles and solution times are shown in Tables 2 and 3. The angles vary significantly from beam selector to beam selector and for the same beam selector with different resolutions. This variability of performance of the heuristics explored here is likely attributable to the redefinition of the solution space that occurs when the judgment function is made "aware" of dose voxels at the interface region of targeted and avoided structures.

Measuring the quality of the selected angles is not obvious. One measure is of course the value of the judgment function. This information is shown in Table 4.

The judgment values indicate that the 5 mm spacing is too course for the fluence model to adequately address the trade-offs between treating the tumor and not treating the brain stem. The 5 mm spacing so crudely approximates

Table 1. The angle values. The top rows are with 5 mm resolution and the bottom rows are with 3 mm resolution.

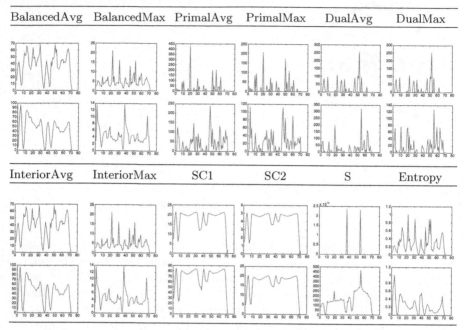

BalancedAvg	BalancedMax	PrimalAvg	PrimalMax	DualAvg	DualMax

InteriorAvg	InteriorMax	SC1	SC2	S	Entropy

the anatomical structures that it was always possible to design a 9-beam treatment that treated the patient as well as a 72-beam treatment. The problem is that the boundaries between target and critical structures, which is where over and under irradiating typically occurs, are not well defined, and hence, the regions that are of most importance are largely ignored. These boundaries are better defined by the 3 mm grid, and a degradation in the judgment value is observed.

Judgment values do not tell the entire story, though, and are only one of many ways to evaluate the quality of treatment plans. The mean judgment values of the different techniques all approach the goal value of -5.0000, and claiming that one technique is better than another based on these values is tenuous. However, there are some outliers, and most significantly the scoring values did poorly with a judgment value of 3.0515 in the scoring and set cover beam selectors. The resulting 3 mm isodose curves and DVH for the scoring 9-beam selector are seen in Figures 8 and 9. These treatments are clearly less than desirable, especially when compared to Figures 4 and 5.

Besides the judgment value, another measure determines how well the selected angles represent the interpretation of the angle values. If we think of the angle values as forming a probability density, then the expected value of the nine selected angles represents the likelihood of the angle collection being optimal. These expected values are found in Table 5.

Table 2. The angles selected by the different beam selectors with 3 mm resolution. The times are in seconds and include the time needed to select angles and design a treatment with these angles.

Selector	Angle Value			Selected Angles						Time
Set Cover	BalancedAvg	15	20	25	55	60	65	70	85	240	113.51
	BalancedMax	10	15	20	95	190	195	200	275	340	126.23
	PrimalAvg	15	125	155	230	235	240	250	300	340	43.96
	PrimalMax	15	25	125	155	170	230	235	250	300	45.52
	DualAvg	10	15	55	95	100	275	295	315	320	34.02
	DualMax	15	55	95	100	110	275	295	315	320	68.80
	InteriorAvg	15	20	25	55	60	65	70	85	240	115.75
	InteriorMax	10	15	20	95	190	195	200	275	340	128.66
	SetCover 1	20	145	150	155	200	320	325	330	335	90.91
	SetCover 2	20	140	145	150	155	200	325	330	335	134.43
	Scoring	245	255	260	265	270	275	280	285	290	108.19
	Entropy	10	15	20	25	55	60	195	200	240	144.43
Scoring	BalancedAvg	15	20	25	55	60	65	70	75	85	104.93
	BalancedMax	10	15	20	25	95	190	195	200	340	108.29
	PrimalAvg	15	125	155	230	235	240	250	300	340	48.59
	PrimalMax	15	25	125	155	170	230	235	250	300	46.22
	DualAvg	10	15	55	95	100	275	295	315	320	36.24
	DualMax	15	55	95	100	110	275	295	315	320	66.56
	InteriorAvg	15	20	25	55	60	65	70	75	85	105.91
	InteriorMax	10	15	20	25	95	190	195	200	340	107.92
	SetCover1	20	145	150	155	200	320	325	330	335	83.87
	SetCover2	20	140	145	150	155	200	325	330	335	104.36
	Scoring	245	255	260	265	270	275	280	285	290	122.59
	Entropy	10	15	20	25	55	60	190	195	200	235.84
VQ	BalancedAvg	30	60	90	120	155	205	255	295	340	197.62
	BalancedMax	20	50	85	130	175	205	245	295	345	71.93
	PrimalAvg	35	90	135	190	235	250	280	320	350	55.27
	PrimalMax	20	70	125	160	205	245	275	305	340	121.91
	DualAvg	35	80	115	180	255	280	290	310	345	115.53
	DualMax	35	80	105	155	225	265	290	310	340	126.94
	InteriorAvg	30	60	90	120	155	205	255	295	340	198.43
	InteriorMax	20	50	85	130	175	205	245	295	345	71.98
	SetCover1	40	75	115	150	190	225	265	300	340	52.56
	SetCover2	40	75	110	145	185	230	265	300	340	187.10
	Scoring	50	95	135	185	230	260	285	305	340	134.33
	Entropy	15	40	65	90	130	175	220	275	340	56.14

The trend to observe is that the set cover and scoring techniques select angles with higher expected values than the vector quantization technique, meaning that the angles selected more accurately represent the intent of the angle values. This is not surprising, as the set cover and scoring methods can be interpreted as attempting to maximize their expected value. However, if

Table 3. The angles selected by the different beam selectors with 5 mm resolution. The times are in seconds and include the time needed to select angles and design a treatment with these angles.

Selector	Angle Value			Selected Angles							Time
Set Cover	BalancedAvg	55	70	75	110	155	250	260	330	335	4.32
	BalancedMax	110	120	155	225	245	250	260	295	300	4.46
	PrimalAvg	45	55	100	150	190	250	260	275	305	4.81
	PrimalMax	45	55	100	150	190	250	260	275	305	4.89
	DualAvg	20	45	110	160	230	250	255	260	275	4.96
	DualMax	20	45	110	160	230	250	255	260	275	5.04
	InteriorAvg	55	70	75	110	155	250	260	330	335	4.67
	InteriorMax	110	120	155	225	245	250	260	295	300	4.90
	SetCover 1	20	145	150	155	200	320	325	330	335	5.43
	SetCover 2	20	140	145	150	155	200	325	330	335	5.79
	Scoring	95	185	230	260	265	270	275	280	320	5.10
	Entropy	70	75	110	155	225	250	260	335	340	5.32
Scoring	BalancedAvg	55	70	75	110	155	250	260	330	335	2.12
	BalancedMax	110	120	155	225	245	250	260	295	300	2.34
	PrimalAvg	45	55	100	150	190	250	260	275	305	2.68
	PrimalMax	45	55	100	150	190	250	260	275	305	2.72
	DualAvg	20	45	110	160	230	250	255	260	275	2.88
	DualMax	20	45	110	160	230	250	255	260	275	2.94
	InteriorAvg	55	70	75	110	155	250	260	330	335	2.48
	InteriorMax	110	120	155	225	245	250	260	295	300	2.78
	SetCover1	20	145	150	155	200	320	325	330	335	3.31
	SetCover2	20	140	145	150	155	200	325	330	335	3.53
	Scoring	95	185	230	260	265	270	275	280	320	3.01
	Entropy	70	75	110	155	225	250	260	335	340	3.24
VQ	BalancedAvg	40	75	105	140	185	230	270	305	345	3.77
	BalancedMax	40	80	115	145	190	235	270	300	340	3.41
	PrimalAvg	40	85	105	130	175	225	265	290	330	3.32
	PrimalMax	30	80	105	130	175	225	260	270	320	4.11
	DualAvg	20	75	130	160	205	245	260	265	315	3.99
	DualMax	20	75	130	160	205	245	260	265	315	4.11
	InteriorAvg	40	75	105	140	185	230	270	305	345	4.40
	InteriorMax	40	80	115	145	190	235	270	300	340	4.03
	SetCover1	40	75	110	145	185	225	265	300	340	4.70
	SetCover2	40	75	110	145	185	230	265	300	340	4.88
	Scoring	185	190	195	200	240	280	285	290	330	5.58
	Entropy	45	75	105	140	195	240	270	305	345	4.75

the angle assignments do not accurately gauge the intrinsic value of an angle, such accuracy is misleading. As an example, both the set cover and scoring methods have an expected value of 1 with respect to the scoring angle values in the 5 mm case. In this case, the only angles with nonzero values are 185

Table 4. The judgment values of the selected angles.

	SC		S		VQ			
	3 mm	5 mm	3 mm	5 mm	3 mm	5 mm	3 mm	Mean
BalancedAvg	-5.0000	-5.0000	-5.0000	-5.0000	-4.9194	-5.0000		-4.9731
BalancedMax	-4.8977	-5.0000	-4.8714	-5.0000	-5.0000	-5.0000		-4.9230
PrimalAvg	-5.0000	-5.0000	-5.0000	-5.0000	-5.0000	-5.0000		-5.0000
PrimalMax	-5.0000	-5.0000	-5.0000	-5.0000	-5.0000	-5.0000		-5.0000
DualAvg	-5.0000	-5.0000	-5.0000	-5.0000	-3.5214	-5.0000		-4.5071
DualMax	-5.0000	-5.0000	-5.0000	-5.0000	-4.8909	-5.0000		-4.9636
InteriorAvg	-5.0000	-5.0000	-5.0000	-5.0000	-4.9194	-5.0000		-4.9731
InteriorMax	-4.8977	-5.0000	-4.8714	-5.0000	-5.0000	-5.0000		-4.9230
SC1	-4.9841	-5.0000	-4.9841	-5.0000	-5.0000	-5.0000		-4.9894
SC2	-4.9820	-5.0000	-4.9820	-5.0000	-4.9984	-5.0000		-4.9875
S	3.0515	-5.0000	3.0515	-5.0000	-4.9967	-5.0000		0.3688
Entropy	-5.0000	-5.0000	-5.0000	-5.0000	-5.0000	-5.0000		-5.0000
Mean	-4.3092	-5.0000	-4.3048	-5.0000	-4.8538	-5.0000		

Table 5. The expected values of the selected angles.

	SC		S		VQ	
	3 mm	5 mm	3 mm	5 mm	3 mm	5 mm
BalancedAvg	0.2157	0.2059	0.2176	0.2059	0.1506	0.1189
BalancedMax	0.2613	0.3045	0.2673	0.3045	0.1234	0.1344
PrimalAvg	0.4191	0.8189	0.4191	0.8189	0.1600	0.0487
PrimalMax	0.4194	0.7699	0.4194	0.7699	0.1362	0.0429
DualAvg	0.6144	0.7443	0.6144	0.7443	0.0394	0.3207
DualMax	0.5264	0.7443	0.5264	0.7443	0.0359	0.3207
InteriorAvg	0.2157	0.2059	0.2176	0.2059	0.1506	0.1189
InteriorMax	0.2613	0.3045	0.2673	0.3045	0.1234	0.1344
SC1	0.1492	0.1461	0.1492	0.1461	0.1251	0.1248
SC2	0.1523	0.1491	0.1523	0.1491	0.1234	0.1273
S	0.2352	1.0000	0.2352	1.0000	0.1673	0.5058
Entropy	0.3176	0.3320	0.3303	0.332	0.1399	0.1402

and 275, and the perfect expected value only indicates that these two angles are selected. A scoring technique that only scores 2 of the 72 possible angles is not meaningful, and in fact, the other 7 angles could be selected at random.

The expected values in Table 5 highlight how the angle assignments differ in philosophy. The weakly informed angle values attempt to measure each angle's individual worth in an optimal treatment, regardless of which other angles are selected. The informed values allow the individual angles to compete through the optimization process for high values, and hence, these values are tempered with the knowledge that other angles will be used. The trend in Table 5 is that informed expected values are lower than weakly informed values, although this is not a perfect correlation.

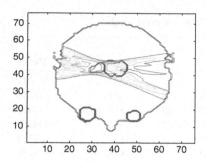

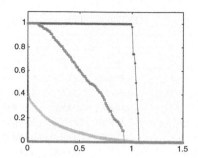

Fig. 8. The 3 mm isodose contours for the balanced treatment when 9 angles were selected with a scoring method and scoring angle values.

Fig. 9. The 3 mm DVH for the balanced treatment when 9 angles were selected with a scoring method and scoring angle values.

From the previous discussions, it is clear that beam selectors depend on the dose point resolution, but none of this discussion attempts to quantify the difference. We conclude with such an attempt. For each of the selected sets of angles, we calculated (in degrees) the difference between consecutive angles. These distances provide a measure of how the angles are spread around the great circle without a concern about specific angles. These values were compared in the 3 mm and 5 mm cases. For example, the nine angles selected by the VQ selector with the BalancedAvg angle values were $\{30, 60, 90, 120, 155, 205, 255, 295, 340\}$ and $\{40, 75, 105, 140, 185, 230, 270, 305, 345\}$ for the 3 mm and 5 mm cases, respectively. The associated relative spacings are $\{30, 30, 30, 35, 50, 50, 40, 45, 50\}$ and $\{35, 30, 35, 45, 45, 40, 35, 40, 55\}$. This information allows us to ask whether or not one set of angles can be rotated to obtain the other. We begin by taking the absolute value of the corresponding relative spacings, so for this example the differences are

$$
\begin{array}{l}
\text{3 mm Relative Spacing } 30 \ 30 \ 30 \ 35 \ 50 \ 50 \ 40 \ 45 \ 50 \\
\underline{\text{5 mm Relative Spacing } 35 \ 30 \ 35 \ 45 \ 45 \ 40 \ 35 \ 40 \ 55} \\
\hspace{2.2cm} \text{Difference } \ 5 \ \ 0 \ \ 5 \ 10 \ \ 5 \ 10 \ \ 5 \ \ 5 \ \ 5
\end{array}
$$

Depending on how the angles from the 3 mm and 5 mm cases interlace, we rotate (or shift) the first set to either the left or the right and repeat the calculation. In our example, the first angle in the 3 mm selection is 30, which is positioned between angles 40 and 345 in the 5 mm case. So we shift the 3 mm relative spacings to the left to obtain the following differences (notice that the first 30 of the 3 mm above is now compared to the last 55 of the 5 mm case).

$$
\begin{array}{l}
\text{3 mm Relative Spacing } 30 \ 30 \ 35 \ 50 \ 50 \ 40 \ 45 \ 50 \ 30 \\
\underline{\text{5 mm Relative Spacing } 35 \ 30 \ 35 \ 45 \ 45 \ 40 \ 35 \ 40 \ 55} \\
\hspace{2.2cm} \text{Difference } \ 5 \ \ 0 \ \ 0 \ \ 5 \ \ 5 \ \ 0 \ 10 \ 10 \ 25
\end{array}
$$

Table 6. The mean and standard deviation of the (minimum) difference between the 3 mm and 5 mm cases.

	Mean			Variance		
	SC	S	VQ	SC	S	VQ
BalancedAvg	45.56	47.78	5.55	2465.30	4706.90	9.03
BalancedMax	40.00	45.56	11.11	2125.00	3346.50	73.61
PrimalAvg	28.89	28.89	14.44	236.11	236.11	165.28
PrimalMax	16.67	16.67	13.33	325.00	325.00	131.25
DualAvg	37.78	37.78	16.67	1563.20	1563.20	150.00
DualMax	36.67	36.67	15.56	1050.00	1050.00	84.03
InteriorAvg	45.56	47.78	5.56	2465.30	4706.90	9.03
InteriorMax	40.00	45.56	11.11	2125.00	3346.50	73.61
SC1	0.00	0.00	1.11	0.00	0.00	4.86
SC2	0.00	0.00	0.00	0.00	0.00	0.00
S	40.00	40.00	35.56	3481.20	3481.20	1909.00
Entropy	44.44	44.44	13.33	1259.00	1552.80	81.25
Mean	31.30	32.59	11.94	1424.60	2026.30	224.25

The smallest aggregate difference, which is 50 in the first comparisons versus 60 in the second, is used in our calculations. We do not include all possible shifts of the first set because some spatial positioning should be respected, and our calculation honors this by comparing spacing between neighboring angles.

Table 6 contains the means and standard deviations of the relative spacing differences.

A low standard deviation indicates that the selected angles in one case are simply rotated versions of the other. For example, the VQ selector with the InteriorAvg angle values has a low standard deviation of 9.03, which means that we can nearly rotate the 3 mm angles of $\{30, 60, 90, 120, 155, 205, 255, 295, 340\}$ to obtain the 5 mm angles of $\{40, 75, 105, 140, 185, 230, 270, 305, 345\}$. In fact, if we rotate the first set 15 degrees, the average discrepancy is the stated mean value of 5.56. A low mean value but a high standard deviation means that it is possible to rotate the 3 mm angles so that several of the angles nearly match but only at the expense of making the others significantly different. Methods with high mean and standard deviations selected substantially different angles for the 3 mm and 5 mm cases.

The last row of Table 6 lists the column averages. These values lead us to speculate that the VQ techniques are less susceptible to changes in the dose point resolution. We were surprised that the SC1 and SC2 angle values were unaffected by the dose point resolution, and that each corresponding beam selector chose (nearly) the same angles independent of the resolution. In any event, it is clear that the dose point resolution generally affects each of the beam selectors.

Besides the numerical comparisons just described, a basic question is whether or not the beam selectors produce clinically adequate angles. Figures

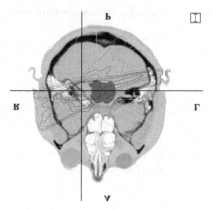

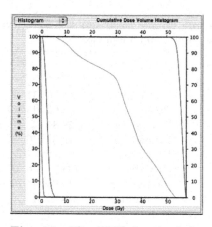

Fig. 10. Isodose contours for initial design of a nine angle clinical treatment plan.

Fig. 11. The DVH for the balanced 72-angle treatment with 5 mm spacing.

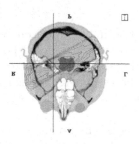

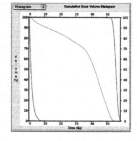

Fig. 12. The isodose contours for a clinically designed treatment based on the 9 angles selected by the set cover method with BalancedAvg angle values and 3 mm spacing.

Fig. 13. The DVH for a clinically designed treatment based on the 9 angles selected by the set cover method with BalancedAvg angle values and 3 mm spacing.

10 and 11 depict the isodose contours and a DVH of a typical clinical 9-angle treatment. This is not necessarily a final treatment plan, but rather what might be typical of an initial estimate of angles to be used. Treatment planners would typically adjust these angles in an attempt to improve the design. Using the BalancedAvg angle values, we used Nomos' commercial software to design the fluence patterns for 9-angle treatments with the angles produced by the three different techniques with 3 mm spacing. Figures 12 through 17 contain the isodose contours and DVHs from the Corvus software.

The set cover and scoring treatment plans in Figures 12 through Figures 15 are clearly inferior to the initial clinical design in that they encroach significantly onto critical structures and normal healthy tissue with high isodose

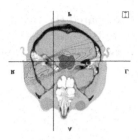

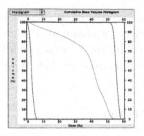

Fig. 14. The isodose contours for a clinically designed treatment based on the 9 angles selected by the scoring method with BalancedAvg angle values and 3 mm spacing.

Fig. 15. The DVH for a clinically designed treatment based on the 9 angles selected by the scoring method with BalancedAvg angle values and 3 mm spacing.

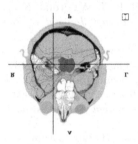

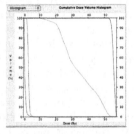

Fig. 16. The isodose contours for a clinically designed treatment based on the 9 angles selected by the vector quantization method with BalancedAvg angle values and 3 mm spacing.

Fig. 17. The DVH for a clinically designed treatment based on the 9 angles selected by the vector quantization method with BalancedAvg angle values and 3 mm spacing. with 5 mm spacing.

levels. The problem is that the 9 angles are selected too close to each other. The fact that these are similar treatments is not surprising since the angle sets only differed by one angle. The vector quantization treatment in Figures 16 and 17 appears to be clinically relevant in that it compares favorably with the initial design of the 9 angle clinical plan (i.e., Figures 10 to 16 comparison and Figures 11 to 17 comparison).

5 Conclusions

We have implemented several heuristic beam selection techniques to investigate the influence of dose grid resolution on these automated beam selection strategies. Testing the heuristics on a clinical case with two different dose point resolutions we have for the first time studied this effect and have found it to be significant. We have also (again for the first time) compared the results with those from a commercial planning system. We believe that the effect of dose grid resolution becomes smaller as resolution increases, but further research is necessary to test that hypothesis.

References

1. R. K. Ahuja and H. W. Hamacher. A network flow algorithm to minimize beam-on-time for unconstrained multileaf collimator problems in cancer radiation therapy. *Networks*, 45:36–41, 2004.
2. D. Baatar, H. W. Hamacher, M. Ehrgott, and G. J. Woeginger. Decomposition of integer matrices and multileaf collimator sequencing. *Discrete Applied Mathematics*, 152:6–34, 2005.
3. T. R. Bortfeld, A. L. Boyer, D. L. Kahler, and T. J. Waldron. X-ray field compensation with multileaf collimators. *International Journal of Radiation Oncology, Biology, Physics*, 28:723–730, 1994.
4. M. Ehrgott, A. Holder, and J. Reese. Beam selection in radiotherapy design. *Linear Algebra and its Applications*, doi: 10.1016/j.laa.2007.05.039, 2007.
5. M. Ehrgott and R. Johnston. Optimisation of beam directions in intensity modulated radiation therapy planning. *OR Spectrum*, 25:251–264, 2003.
6. A. Gersho and R. Gray. *Vector Quantization and Signal Compression*. Kluwer Academic Publishers, Boston, MA, 1991.
7. H. W. Hamacher and K. H. Küfer. Inverse radiation therapy planing – A multiple objective optimization approach. *Discrete Applied Mathematics*, 118: 145–161, 2002.
8. A. Holder. Designing radiotherapy plans with elastic constraints and interior point methods. *Health Care Management Science*, 6:5–16, 2003.
9. A. Holder. Partitioning multiple objective optimal solutions with applications in radiotherapy design. *Optimization and Engineering*, 7:501–526, 2006.
10. A. Holder and B. Salter. A tutorial on radiation oncology and optimization. In H. Greenberg, editor, *Emerging Methodologies and Applications in Operations Research*, chapter 4. Kluwer Academic Press, Boston, MA, 2004.
11. S. Kamath, S. Sahni, J. Li, J. Palta, and S. Ranka. Leaf sequencing algorithms for segmented multileaf collimation. *Physics in Medicine and Biology*, 48:307–324, 2003.
12. P. Kolmonen, J. Tervo, and P. Lahtinen. Use of the Cimmino algorithm and continuous approximation for the dose deposition kernel in the inverse problem of radiation treatment planning. *Physics in Medicine and Biology*, 43:2539–2554, 1998.
13. E. K. Lee, T. Fox, and I. Crocker. Integer programming applied to intensity-modulated radiation therapy treatment planning. *Annals of Operations Research*, 119:165–181, 2003.
14. G. J. Lim, M. C. Ferris, S. J. Wright, D. M. Shepard, and M. A. Earl. An optimization framework for conformal radiation treatment planning. INFORMS *Journal on Computing*, 13:366–380, 2007.
15. J. Löf. *Development of a general framework for optimization of radiation therapy*. PhD thesis, Department of Medical Radiation Physics, Karolinska Institute, Stockholm, Sweden, 2000.

16. S. Morrill, I. Rosen, R. Lane, and J. Belli. The influence of dose constraint point placement on optimized radiation therapy treatment planning. *International Journal of Radiation Oncology, Biology, Physics*, 19:129–141, 1990.

17. P. Nizin, A. Kania, and K. Ayyangar. Basic concepts of corvus dose model. *Medical Dosimetry*, 26:65–69, 2001.

18. P. Nizin and R. Mooij. An approximation of central-axis absorbed dose in narrow photon beams. *Medical Physics*, 24:1775–1780, 1997.

19. F. Preciado-Walters, R. Rardin, M. Langer, and V. Thai. A coupled column generation, mixed integer approach to optimal planning of intensity modulated radiation therapy for cancer. *Mathematical Programming*, 101:319–338, 2004.

20. A. Pugachev and L. Xing. Pseudo beam's-eye-view as applied to beam orientation selection in intensity-modulated radiation therapy. *International Journal of Radiation Oncology, Biology, Physics*, 51:1361–1370, 2001.

21. H. E. Romeijn, R. K. Ahuja, J. F. Dempsey, A. Kumar, and J. G. Li. A novel linear programming approach to fluence map optimization for intensity modulated radiation therapy treatment planning. *Physics in Medicine and Biology*, 48:3521–3542, 2003.

22. H. E. Romeijn, J. F. Dempsey, and J. G. Li. A unifying framework for multicriteria fluence map optimization models. *Physics in Medicine and Biology*, 49:1991–2013, 2004.

23. I. J. Rosen, R. G. Lane, S. M. Morrill, and J. Belli. Treatment planning optimisation using linear programming. *Medical Physics*, 18:141–152, 1991.

24. W. Schlegel and A. Mahr. *3D-Conformal Radiation Therapy: A Multimedia Introduction to Methods and Techniques*. Springer Verlag, Heidelberg, 2002. Springer Verlag, Berlin.

25. R. A. C. Siochi. Minimizing static intensity modulation delivery time using an intensity solid paradigm. *International Journal of Radiation Oncology, Biology, Physics*, 43:671–689, 1999.

26. S. Söderström and A. Brahme. Selection of beam orientations in radiation therapy using entropy and fourier transform measures. *Physics in Medicine and Biology*, 37:911–924, 1992.

27. S. V. Spirou and C. S. Chui. A gradient inverse planning algorithm with dose-volume constraints. *Medical Physics*, 25:321–333, 1998.

28. C. Wang, J. Dai, and Y. Hu. Optimization of beam orientations and beam weights for conformal radiotherapy using mixed integer programming. *Physics in Medicine and Biology*, 48:4065–4076, 2003.

29. S. Webb. *Intensity-modulated radiation therapy (Series in Medical Physics)*. Institute of Physics Publishing, 2001.

30. I. Winz. A decision support system for radiotherapy treatment planning. Master's thesis, Department of Engineering Science, School of Engineering, University of Auckland, New Zealand, 2004.

31. P. Xia and L. Verhey. Multileaf collimator leaf sequencing algorithm for intensity modulated beams with multiple segments. *Medical Physics*, 25:1424–1434, 1998.

Decomposition of matrices and static multileaf collimators: a survey

Matthias Ehrgott[1*], Horst W. Hamacher[2†], and Marc Nußbaum[2]

[1] Department of Engineering Science, The University of Auckland, Auckland, New Zealand. m.ehrgott@auckland.ac.nz
[2] Fachbereich Mathematik, Technische Universität Kaiserslautern, Kaiserslautern, Germany. hamacher@mathematik.uni-kl.de

Summary. Multileaf Collimators (MLC) consist of (currently 20-100) pairs of movable metal leaves which are used to block radiation in Intensity Modulated Radiation Therapy (IMRT). The leaves modulate a uniform source of radiation to achieve given intensity profiles. The modulation process is modeled by the decomposition of a given non-negative integer matrix into a non-negative linear combination of matrices with the (strict) consecutive ones property.

In this paper we review some results and algorithms which can be used to minimize the time a patient is exposed to radiation (corresponding to the sum of coefficients in the linear combination), the set-up time (corresponding to the number of matrices used in the linear combination), and other objectives which contribute to an improved radiation therapy.

Keywords: Intensity modulated radiation therapy, multileaf collimator, intensity map segmentation, complexity, multi objective optimization.

1 Introduction

Intensity modulated radiation therapy (IMRT) is a form of cancer therapy which has been used since the beginning of the 1990s. Its success in fighting cancer is based on the fact that it can modulate radiation, taking specific patient data into consideration. Mathematical optimization has contributed considerably since the end of the 1990s (see, for instance, [31]) concentrating mainly on three areas,

---

* The research has been partially supported by University of Auckland Researcher's Strategic Support Initiative grant 360875/9275.

† The research has been partially supported by Deutsche Forschungsgemeinschaft (DFG) grant HA 1737/7 "Algorithmik großer und komplexer Netzwerke" and by New Zealand's Julius von Haast Award.

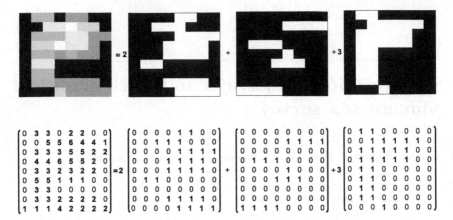

$$
\begin{bmatrix}
0 & 3 & 3 & 0 & 2 & 2 & 0 & 0\\
0 & 0 & 5 & 5 & 6 & 4 & 4 & 1\\
0 & 3 & 3 & 3 & 5 & 5 & 2 & 2\\
0 & 4 & 4 & 6 & 5 & 5 & 2 & 0\\
0 & 3 & 3 & 2 & 3 & 2 & 2 & 0\\
0 & 5 & 5 & 1 & 1 & 1 & 0 & 0\\
0 & 3 & 3 & 0 & 0 & 0 & 0 & 0\\
0 & 3 & 3 & 2 & 2 & 2 & 2 & 0\\
1 & 1 & 1 & 4 & 2 & 2 & 2 & 2
\end{bmatrix}
= 2
\begin{bmatrix}
0 & 0 & 0 & 0 & 1 & 1 & 0 & 0\\
0 & 0 & 1 & 1 & 1 & 0 & 0 & 0\\
0 & 0 & 0 & 0 & 1 & 1 & 1 & 1\\
0 & 0 & 0 & 1 & 1 & 1 & 1 & 0\\
0 & 0 & 0 & 1 & 1 & 1 & 1 & 0\\
0 & 1 & 1 & 0 & 0 & 0 & 0 & 0\\
0 & 0 & 0 & 0 & 0 & 0 & 0 & 0\\
0 & 0 & 0 & 1 & 1 & 1 & 1 & 0\\
0 & 0 & 0 & 0 & 1 & 1 & 1 & 1
\end{bmatrix}
+
\begin{bmatrix}
0 & 0 & 0 & 0 & 0 & 0 & 0 & 0\\
0 & 0 & 0 & 0 & 1 & 1 & 1 & 1\\
0 & 0 & 0 & 0 & 0 & 0 & 0 & 0\\
0 & 1 & 1 & 1 & 0 & 0 & 0 & 0\\
0 & 0 & 0 & 0 & 1 & 0 & 0 & 0\\
0 & 0 & 0 & 1 & 1 & 1 & 0 & 0\\
0 & 0 & 0 & 0 & 0 & 0 & 0 & 0\\
0 & 0 & 0 & 0 & 0 & 0 & 0 & 0\\
1 & 1 & 1 & 1 & 0 & 0 & 0 & 0
\end{bmatrix}
+3
\begin{bmatrix}
0 & 1 & 1 & 0 & 0 & 0 & 0 & 0\\
0 & 0 & 1 & 1 & 1 & 1 & 1 & 0\\
0 & 1 & 1 & 1 & 1 & 1 & 0 & 0\\
0 & 1 & 1 & 1 & 1 & 1 & 0 & 0\\
0 & 1 & 1 & 0 & 0 & 0 & 0 & 0\\
0 & 1 & 1 & 0 & 0 & 0 & 0 & 0\\
0 & 1 & 1 & 0 & 0 & 0 & 0 & 0\\
0 & 1 & 1 & 0 & 0 & 0 & 0 & 0\\
0 & 0 & 0 & 1 & 0 & 0 & 0 & 0
\end{bmatrix}
$$

Fig. 1. Realization of an intensity matrix by overlaying radiation fields with different MLC segments.

- the geometry problem,
- the intensity problem, and
- the realization problem.

The first of these problems finds the best selection of radiation angles, i.e., the angles from which radiation is delivered. A recent paper with the most up to date list of references for this problem can be found in [17]. Once a solution of the geometry problem has been found, an *intensity profile* is determined for each of the angles. These intensity profiles can be found, for instance, with the multicriteria approach of [20] or many other intensity optimization methods (see [30] for more references). In Figure 1, an intensity profile is shown as greyscale coded grid. We assume that the intensity profile has been discretized such that the different shades in this grid can be represented by non-negative integers, where black corresponds to 0 and larger integers are used for lighter colors. In the following we will therefore think of intensity profiles and $N \times M$ *intensity matrices* A as one and the same.

In this paper, we assume that solutions for the geometry and intensity problems have been found and focus on the problem of realizing the intensity matrix A using so-called (static) *multileaf collimators* (*MLC*). Radiation is blocked by M (left, right) pairs of metal leaves, each of which can be positioned between the cells of the corresponding intensity profile. The opening corresponding to a cell of the segment is referred to as a bixel or beamlet. On the right-hand-side of Figure 1, three possible *segments* for the intensity profile on the left of Figure 1 are shown, where the black areas in the three rectangles correspond to the left and right leaves. Radiation passes (perpendicular to the plane represented by the segments) through the opening between the leaves (white areas). The goal is to find a set of MLC segments such that the intensity matrix A is realized by irradiating each of these segments for a certain amount of time (2, 1, and 3 in Figure 1).

In the same way as intensity profiles and integer matrices correspond to each other, each segment in Figure 1 can be represented by a binary $M \times N$ matrix $Y = (y_{mn})$, where $y_{mn} = 1$ if and only if radiation can pass through bixel (m, n). Since the area left open by each pair of leaves is contiguous, the matrix Y possesses the (strict) *consecutive-ones (C1)* property in its rows, i.e., for all $m \in \mathcal{M} := \{1, \dots, M\}$ and $n \in \mathcal{N} := \{1, \dots, N\}$ there exists a pair $l_m \in \mathcal{N}, r_m \in \mathcal{N} \cup \{N + 1\}$ such that

$$y_{mn} = 1 \iff l_m \leq n < r_m. \tag{1}$$

Hence the realization problem can be formulated as the following *C1 decomposition problem*. Let $\mathcal{K}$ be the index set of all $M \times N$ consecutive-ones matrices and let $\mathcal{K}' \subseteq \mathcal{K}$. A *C1 decomposition* (with respect to $\mathcal{K}'$) is defined by non-negative integers $\alpha_k, k \in \mathcal{K}'$ and $M \times N$ C1 matrices $Y^k, k \in \mathcal{K}'$ such that

$$A = \sum_{k \in \mathcal{K}'} \alpha_k Y^k. \tag{2}$$

The coefficients α_k are often called the *monitor units, MU,* of Y^k. In order to evaluate the quality of a C1 decomposition various objective functions have been used in the literature.

The beam-on-time (BOT), total number of monitor units, or *decomposition time (DT)* objective

$$DT(\alpha) := \sum_{k \in \mathcal{K}'} \alpha_k \tag{3}$$

is a measure for the time a patient is exposed to radiation. Since every change from one segment of the MLC to another takes time, the number of segments or *decomposition cardinality (DC)*

$$DC(\alpha) := |\{\alpha_k : \alpha_k > 0\}| \tag{4}$$

is used to evaluate the (constant) *set-up time*

$$SU_{const}(\alpha) := \tau DC(\alpha) \tag{5}$$

for the MLC. Here we assume that it takes constant time τ to move from one segment to the next. If, on the other hand, τ_{kl} is a variable time to move from Y^k to Y^l and $Y^1, \dots, Y^K$ are the C1 matrices used in a decomposition, then one can also consider the *variable set-up time*

$$SU_{var}(\alpha) = \sum_{k=1}^{K-1} \tau_{\pi(k),\pi(k+1)}. \tag{6}$$

Obviously, this objective depends on the sequence $\pi(1), \dots, \pi(K)$ of these C1 matrices. The *treatment time* is finally defined for each radiation angle by

$$TT(\alpha) := DT(\alpha) + SU(\alpha), \tag{7}$$

where $SU(\alpha) \in \{SU_{var}(\alpha), SU_{const}(\alpha)\}$. Since the set-up time $SU(\alpha)$ can be of the constant or variable kind, two different definitions of treatment time are possible.

For therapeutic and economic reasons, it is desirable to find decompositions with small beam-on, set-up, and treatment times. These will be the optimization problems considered in the subsequent sections.

In this paper we will summarize some basic results and present the ideas of algorithms to solve the decomposition time (Section 2) and the decomposition cardinality (Section 3) problem. In Section 4 we will deal with combined objective functions and mention some current research questions.

2 Algorithms for the decomposition time problem

In this section we consider a given $M \times N$ non-negative integer matrix A corresponding to an intensity profile and look for the decomposition (2) of A into a non-negative linear combination $A = \sum_{k \in \mathcal{K}'} \alpha_k Y^k$ of C1 matrices such that the decomposition time (3) $DT(\alpha) := \sum_{k \in \mathcal{K}'} \alpha_k$ is minimized. First, we review results of the *unconstrained DT problem* in which all C1 matrices can be used, i.e., $\mathcal{K}' = \mathcal{K}$. Then we discuss the *constrained DT problem*, where technical requirements exclude certain C1 matrices, i.e., $\mathcal{K}' \subsetneq \mathcal{K}$.

2.1 Unconstrained DT problem

The most important argument in the unconstrained case is the fact that it suffices to solve the DT problem for single row matrices.

Lemma 1. $A = \sum_{k \in \mathcal{K}} \alpha_k Y^k$ *is a decomposition with decomposition time* $DT(\alpha) := \sum_{k \in \mathcal{K}} \alpha_k$ *if and only if each row* A_m *of* A *has a decomposition* $A_m = \sum_{k \in \mathcal{K}} \alpha_{k_m} Y_m^k$ *into C1 row matrices with decomposition time* $DT(\alpha_m) := \sum_{k \in \mathcal{K}} \alpha_{k_m}$, *such that*

$$DT(\alpha) := \max_{m=1}^{M} DT(\alpha_m). \tag{8}$$

The proof of this result follows from the fact that in the unconstrained DT problem, the complete set of all C1 matrices can be used. Hence, the decomposition of the row with largest $DT(\alpha_m)$ can be extended in an arbitrary fashion by decompositions of the other rows to yield a decomposition of the matrix A with $DT(\alpha) = DT(\alpha_m)$.

The most prominent reference in which the insight of Lemma 1 is used is [8], which introduces the *sweep algorithm*. Each row is considered independently and then checked from left to right, if a position of a left or right leaf needs to be changed in order to realize given intensities a_{mn}. While most practitioners agree that the sweep algorithm provides decompositions with short

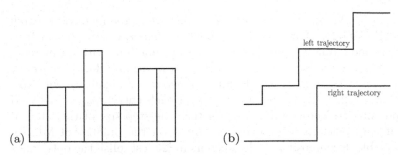

Fig. 2. Representation of intensity row $A_m = (2, 3, 3, 5, 2, 2, 4, 4)$ by rods (a) and the corresponding left and right trajectories (b).

$DT(\alpha)$, the optimality of the algorithm was only proved several years later. We will review some of the papers containing proofs below.

An algorithm which is quoted very often in the MLC optimization literature is that of [32]. Each entry a_{mn} of the intensity map is assigned to a *rod*, the length of which represents the value a_{mn} (see Figure 2). The standard step-and-shoot approach, which is shared by all static MLC algorithms, is implemented in two parts, the *rod pushing* and the *extraction*. While the objective in [32] is to minimize total treatment time TT_{var}, the proposed algorithm is only guaranteed to find a solution that minimizes $DT(\alpha)$.

The authors in [1] prove the optimality of the sweep algorithm by transforming the DT problem into a linear program. The decomposition of a row A_m into C1 row-matrices is first reformulated in a transposed form, i.e., the column vector A_m^T is decomposed into C1 column-matrices (columns with 1s in a single block). This yields a linear system of equations, where the columns of the coefficient matrix are all possible $N(N-1)/2$ C1 column-matrices, the variables are the (unknown) decomposition times and the right-hand-side vector is the transpose A_m^T of row A_m. The objective of the linear program is the sum of the MUs. Such a linear program is well known (see [2]) to be equivalent to a network flow problem in a network with N nodes and $N(N-1)/2$ arcs. The authors in [1] use the special structure of the network and present a shortest augmenting path algorithm which saturates at least one of the nodes in each iteration. Since each of the paths can be constructed in constant time, the complexity for computing $DT(\alpha_m)$ is $\mathcal{O}(N)$. This algorithm is applied to each of the rows of A, such that Lemma 1 implies the following result.

Theorem 1 ([1]). *The unconstrained decomposition time problem for a given non-negative integer $M \times N$ matrix A can be solved in $\mathcal{O}(NM)$ time.*

It is important to notice that the identification of the flow augmenting path and the determination of the flow value which is sent along this path can be interpreted as the two phases of the step-and-shoot process in the sweep algorithm of [8], thus establishing its optimality.

An alternative optimality proof of the sweep algorithm can be found in [23]. Their methodology is based on analyzing the *left and right leaf trajectories* for each row $A_m, m \in \mathcal{M}$. These trajectory functions are at the focus of research in dynamic MLC models. For static MLC in which each leaf moves from left to right, they are monotonously non-decreasing step functions with an increase of $|a_{m,n+1} - a_{m,n}|$ in the left or right trajectory at position n if $a_{m,n+1} - a_{m,n}$ increases or decreases, respectively. Figure 2 illustrates an example with row $A_m = (2, 3, 3, 5, 2, 2, 4, 4)$, the representation of each entry a_{mn} as *rod*, and the corresponding trajectories. By proving that the step size of the left leaf trajectory in any position n is an upper bound on the number of MUs of any other feasible decompositions, the authors in [23] establish the optimality of the decomposition delivered by their algorithm SINGLEPAIR for the case of single row DT problems. In combination with Lemma 1, this yields the optimality of their solution algorithm MULTIPAIR for the unconstrained DT problem, which is, again, a validity proof of the sweep algorithm.

The same bounding argument as in [23] is used by the author in [18] in his TNMU algorithm (*total number of monitor units*). Instead of using trajectories, he bases his work directly on the $M \times (N + 1)$ *difference matrix*

$$D = (d_{mn}) \text{ with } d_{mn} := a_{mn} - a_{m(n-1)}$$
$$\text{for all } m = 1, \ldots, M, n = 1, \ldots, N + 1. \tag{9}$$

Here, $a_{m0} := a_{m(n+1)} := 0$. In each iteration, the TNMU algorithm reduces the *TNMU complexity of A*

$$C(A) := \max_{m \in \mathcal{M}} C_m(A), \tag{10}$$

where $C_m(A) := \sum_{n=1}^{N+1} \max\{0, d_{m,n}\}$ is the *row complexity* of row A_m. More precisely, in each iteration the algorithm identifies some integer $p > 0$ and some C1 matrix Y such that $A' = A - pY$ has non-negative entries and its TNMU complexity satisfies $C(A') = C(A) - p$. Various strategies are recommended to find suitable p and Y, one version of which results in an $\mathcal{O}(N^2 M^2)$ algorithm. As a consequence of its proof, the following closed form expression for the optimal objective value of the DT problem in terms of the TNMU complexity is attained.

Theorem 2 ([18]). *The unconstrained decomposition time problem for a given non-negative integer $M \times N$ matrix A has optimal objective value $DT(\alpha) = C(A)$.*

As will be seen in Section 3.2, this idea also leads to algorithms for the decomposition cardinality problem.

2.2 Constrained DT problem

Depending on the type of MLC, several restrictions may apply to the choice of C1 matrices Y^k which are used in decomposition (2), i.e. $\mathcal{K}' \subsetneq \mathcal{K}$. For example, the mechanics of the multileaf collimator may require that left and right leaf pairs (l_{m-1}, r_{m-1}) and (l_m, r_m) in adjacent rows Y_{m-1} and Y_m of any C1 matrix Y must not overlap (*interleaf motion constraints*). More specifically, we call a C1 matrix Y *shape matrix* if

$$l_{m-1} \leq r_m \text{ and } r_{m-1} \geq l_m \tag{11}$$

holds for all $m = 2, \ldots, M$. The matrix

$$Y = \begin{pmatrix} 0 & 1 & 1 & 0 & 0 & 0 & 0 \\ 0 & 0 & 0 & 0 & 1 & 1 & 0 \\ 0 & 0 & 1 & 1 & 1 & 0 & 0 \\ 1 & 0 & 0 & 0 & 0 & 0 & 0 \end{pmatrix}$$

is, for instance, a C1 matrix, but not a shape matrix, since there are two violations of (11), namely $r_1 = 4 < 5 = l_2$ and $l_3 = 3 > 2 = r_4$. By drawing the left and right leaves corresponding to the left and right sets of zeros in each row of Y, it is easy to understand why the constraints (11) are called interleaf motion constraints.

Another important restriction is the *width* or *innerleaf motion* constraint

$$r_m - l_m \geq \delta \text{ for all } m \in \mathcal{M}, \tag{12}$$

where $\delta > 0$ is a given (integer) constant.

A final constraint may be enforced to control *tongue-and-groove* (*T&G*) *error* which often makes the decomposition model (2) inaccurate. Since several MLC types have T&G joints between adjacent leaf pairs, the thinner material in the tongue and the groove causes a smaller or larger radiation than predicted in model 2 if a leaf covers bixel m, n (i.e., $y_{mn} = 0$), but not $m+1, n$ (i.e., $y_{m+1,n} = 1$), or vice versa. Some of this error is unavoidable, but a decomposition with $y_{mn}^k = 1, y_{m+1,n}^k = 0$ and $y_{mn}^{k'} = 0, y_{m+1,n}^{k'} = 1$ can often be avoided by swapping the mth rows of Y^k and $Y^{k'}$.

The authors in [7] present a polynomial algorithm for the DT problem with interleaf motion and width constraints by reducing it to a network flow problem with side constraints. They first construct a layered graph $G = (V, E)$, the *shape matrix graph* which has M layers of nodes. The nodes in each layer represent left-right leaf set-ups in an MLC satisfying the width constraint or — equivalently — a feasible row in a shape matrix (see Figure 3). More precisely, node (m, l, r) stands for a possible row m in a C1 matrix with left leaf in position l and right leaf in position r, where the width constraint is modeled by allowing only nodes (m, l, r) with $r - l \geq \delta$. Hence, in each layer there are $\mathcal{O}(N(N-1))$ nodes, and the network has $\mathcal{O}(MN^2)$ nodes. Interleaf motion constraints are modeled by the definition of the arc set E according to $((m, l, r), (m+1, l', r')) \in E$ if and only if $r' - l \geq \delta$ and $r - l' \geq \delta$.

It should be noted that the definition of the arcs can also be adapted to include the *extended interleaf motion constraint*

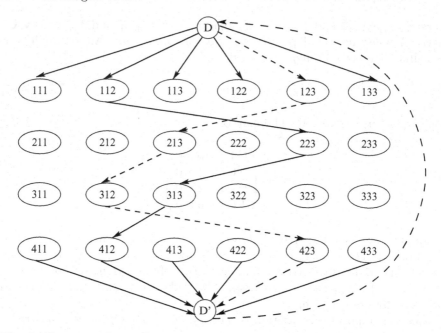

Fig. 3. Shape matrix graph with two paths corresponding to two shape matrices. (Both paths are extended by the return arc (D', D).)

$$r_m - l_{m-1} \geq \gamma \text{ and } l_m - r_{m-1} \geq \gamma \text{ for all } m \in \mathcal{M}, \tag{13}$$

where $\gamma > 0$ is a given (integer) constant. Also, T&G constraints can be modeled by the network structure. If we add a supersource D and a supersink D' connected to all nodes $(1, l, r)$ of the first layer and from all nodes (M, l, r) of the last layer, respectively (see Figure 3), the following result is easy to show.

Lemma 2 ([7]). *Matrix Y with rows $y_1, \ldots, y_M$ is a shape matrix satisfying width (with respect to given δ) and extended interleaf motion (with respect to given γ) constraints if and only if $P(Y)$ is a path from D to D' in G where node (m, l, r) in layer m corresponds to row m of matrix Y.*

In the example of Figure 3 the two paths correspond to the two shape matrices

$$Y^k = \begin{pmatrix} 1 & 0 \\ 0 & 1 \\ 1 & 1 \\ 1 & 0 \end{pmatrix} \text{ and } Y^{k'} = \begin{pmatrix} 0 & 1 \\ 1 & 1 \\ 1 & 0 \\ 0 & 1 \end{pmatrix}.$$

Since paths in the shape matrix graph are in one-to-one correspondence with shape matrices, the scalar multiplication $\alpha_k Y^k$ in decomposition (2) is equivalent to sending α_k units of flow along path P_{Y^k} from D to D'. Hence, the DT problem is equivalent to a network flow problem.

Theorem 3 ([7]). *The decomposition time problem with respect to a given non-negative integer valued matrix A is equivalent to the decomposition network flow problem: Minimize the flow value from source D to sink D' subject to the constraints that for all m ∈ $\mathcal{M}$ and n ∈ $\mathcal{N}$, the sum of the flow through nodes (m, l, r) with $l \leq n < r$ equals the entry $a_{m,n}$. In particular, the DT problem is solvable in polynomial time.*

The polynomiality of the decomposition network flow algorithm follows, since it is a special case of a linear program. Its computation times are very short, but it generally produces a non-integer set of decomposition times as solution, while integrality is for various practical reasons a highly desirable feature in any decomposition. The authors in [7] show that there always exists an alternative integer solution, which can, in fact, be obtained by a modification of the shape matrix graph. This version of the network flow approach is, however, not numerically competitive.

An improved network flow formulation is given by [4]. A smaller network is used with $\mathcal{O}(MN)$ nodes instead of the shape matrix graph G with $\mathcal{O}(MN^2)$ nodes. This is achieved by replacing each layer of G by two sets of nodes, representing a potential left and right leaf position, respectively. An arc between two of these nodes represents a row of a C1 matrix. The resulting linear programming formulation has a coefficient matrix which can be shown to be totally unimodular, such that the linear program yields an integer solution. Numerical experiments show that this double layer approach improves the running time of the algorithm considerably.

In [5] a further step is taken by formulating a sequence of integer programs, each of which can be solved by a combinatorial algorithm, i.e., does not require any linear programming solver. The variables in these integer programs correspond to the incremental increases in decomposition time which are caused by the interleaf motion constraint. Using arguments from multicriteria optimization, the following complexity result shows that compared with the unconstrained case of Theorem 1, the complexity only worsens by a factor of M.

Theorem 4 ([5]). *The constrained decomposition time problem with (extended) interleaf and width constraint can be solved in $\mathcal{O}(NM^2)$ time.*

While the preceding approaches maintain the constraints throughout the course of the algorithm, [23, 24] solve the constrained decomposition time problem by starting with a solution of the unconstrained problem. If this solution satisfies all constraints it is obviously optimal. If the optimal solution violates the width constraint, there does not exist a solution which does. Violations of interleaf motion and tongue-and-groove constraints are eliminated by a bounded number of modification steps. A similar correction approach is taken by [32] starting from his rod-pushing and extraction algorithm for the unconstrained case.

In the paper of [22] the idea of the unconstrained algorithm of [18] is carried over to the case of interleaf motion constraints. First, a linear program (LP) is formulated with constraints (2). Hence, the LP has an exponential number of variables. Its dual is solved by a maximal path problem in an acyclic graph. The optimal dual objective value is proved to correspond to a feasible C1 decomposition, i.e., a primally feasible solution of the LP, thus establishing the optimality of the decomposition using the strong LP duality theorem.

3 Algorithms for the decomposition cardinality problem

3.1 Complexity of the DC problem

In contrast to the decomposition time problem, we cannot expect an efficient algorithm which solves the decomposition cardinality problem exactly.

Theorem 5. *The decomposition cardinality problem is strongly NP-hard even in the unconstrained case. In particular, the following results hold.*

1. *[5] The DC problem is strongly NP-hard for matrices with a single row.*
2. *[14] The DC problem is strongly NP-hard for matrices with a single column.*

The first NP-hardness proof for the DC problem is due to [9], who shows that the subset sum problem can be reduced to the DC problem. His proof applies to the case of matrices A with at least two rows. Independently, the authors in [12] use the knapsack problem to prove the (non-strong) NP-hardness in the single-row case. The stronger result of Theorem 5 uses a reduction from the 3-partition problem for the single row case. The result for single column matrices uses a reduction from a variant of the satisfiability problem, NAE-3SAT(5).

A special case, for which the DC problem can be solved in polynomial time, is considered in the next result.

Theorem 6 ([5]). *If $A = pB$ is a positive integer multiple of a binary matrix B, then the C1 decomposition cardinality problem can be solved in polynomial time for the constrained and unconstrained case.*

If A is a binary matrix, this result follows from the polynomial solvability of $DT(\alpha)$, since α_k is binary for all $k \in \mathcal{K}'$ and thus $DT(\alpha) = DC(\alpha)$. If $A = pB$ with $p > 1$, it can be shown that the DC problem for A can be reduced to the solution of the DT problem for B.

Theorem 6 is also important in the analysis of the algorithm of [33]. The main idea is to group the decomposition into phases where in phase k, only matrix elements with values $a_{mn} \geq 2^{R-k}$ are considered, i.e., the matrix elements can be represented by ones and zeros depending on whether $a_{mn} \geq 2^k$

or not ($R = \log_2(\max a_{mn})$). By Theorem 6 each of the decomposition cardinality problems can be solved in polynomial time using a DT algorithm.
Hence, the Xia-Verhey algorithm runs in polynomial time and gives the best
decomposition cardinality, but only among all decompositions with the same
separation into phases.

In view of Theorem 5, most of the algorithms in the literature are heuristic
or approximative (with performance guarantee). Most often, they guarantee
minimal $DT(\alpha)$ and minimize $DC(\alpha)$ heuristically or exactly subject to DT
optimality. The few algorithms that are able to solve the problem exactly
have exponential running time and are limited to small instances, as evident
in Section 5.

3.2 Algorithms for the unconstrained DC problem

The author in [18] applies a greedy idea to his TNMU algorithm. In each of
his extraction steps $A' = A - pY$, p is computed as maximal possible value
such that the pair (p, Y) is *admissible*, i.e., $a'_{mn} \geq 0$ for all m, n and $C(A') = C(A) - p$. Since the algorithm is a specialized version of Engel's decomposition
time algorithm, it will only find good decomposition cardinalities among all
optimal solutions of the DT problem. Note, however (see Example 1), that
none of the optimal solutions of the DT problem may be optimal for the DC
problem.

The author in [21] shows the validity of an algorithm which solves the lexi-
cographic problem of finding among all optimizers of DT one with smallest decomposition cardinality DC. The complexity of this algorithm is $\mathcal{O}(MN^{2L+2})$,
i.e., it is polynomial in M and N, but exponential in L (where L is a bound
for the entries a_{mn} of the matrix A). It should be noted that this algorithm
does not, in general, solve DC. This is due to the fact that among the optimal
solutions for DT there may not be an optimal solution for DC (see Sections
4 and 5).

The idea of Kalinowski's algorithm can, however, be extended to solve
DC. The main idea of this approach is to treat the decomposition time as
a parameter c and to solve the problem of finding a decomposition with
smallest cardinality such that its decomposition time is bounded by c. For
$c = \min DT(\alpha)$, this can be done by Kalinowski's algorithm in $\mathcal{O}(MN^{2L+2})$.
For $c = 1, \ldots, MNL$, the author in [28] shows that the complexity increases
to $\mathcal{O}((MN)^{2L+2})$. We thus have the following result.

Theorem 7 ([28]). *The problem of minimizing the decomposition cardinality* $DC(\alpha)$ *in an unconstrained problem can be solved in* $\mathcal{O}((MN)^{2L+3})$.

The authors in [27] present approximation algorithms for the unconstrained DC problem. They define matrices P_k whose elements are the kth
digits in the binary representation of the entries in A. The (easy) segmentation
of P_k for $k = 1, \ldots, \log L$ then results in a $\mathcal{O}(MN \log(L))$ time ($\log\lfloor L \rfloor + 1$)-
approximation algorithm for DC. They show that the performance guarantee

can be improved to $\lfloor \log D \rfloor + 1$ by choosing D as the maximum of a set of numbers containing all absolute differences between any two consecutive row entries over all rows and the first and last entries of each row. In the context of approximation algorithms we finally mention the following result by [6].

Theorem 8. *The DC problem is APX-hard even for matrices with a single row with entries polynomially bounded in N.*

3.3 Algorithms for the constrained DC problem

A similar idea as in [18] is used in [5] for the constrained decomposition cardinality problem. Data from the solution of the DT problem (see Section 2) is used as input for a greedy extraction procedure. The author in [22] also generalizes the idea of Engel to the case of DC problems with interleaf motion constraints.

The authors in [10–13] consider the decomposition cardinality problem with interleaf motion, width, and tongue-and-groove constraints. The first two groups of constraints are considered by a geometric argumentation. The given matrix A is — similar to [32] — interpreted as a 3-dimensional set of rods, or as they call it a *3D-mountain*, where the height of each rod is determined by the value of its corresponding matrix entry a_{mn}. The decomposition is done by a *mountain reduction technique*, where tongue-and-groove constraints are taken into consideration using a graph model. The underlying graph is complete with its node set corresponding to all feasible C1 matrices. The weight of the edges is determined by the tongue-and-groove error occurring if both matrices are used in a decomposition. Matching algorithms are used to minimize the tongue-and-groove error. In order to speed up the algorithm, smaller graphs are used and the optimal matchings are computed using a network flow algorithm in a sparse graph.

The authors in [19] propose a difference-matrix metaheuristic to obtain solutions with small DC as well as small DT values. The metaheuristic uses a multiple start local search with a heuristic that sequentially extracts segments Y_k based on results of [18]. They consider multiple constraints on the segments, including interleaf and innerleaf motion constraints. Reported results clearly outperform the heuristics implemented in the Elekta MLC system.

4 Combined objective functions

A first combination of decomposition time and cardinality problems is the treatment time problem with constant set-up times $TT(\alpha) := DT(\alpha) + SU(\alpha) = DT(\alpha) + \tau DC(\alpha)$. For τ suitably large, it is clear that the DC problem is a special case of the TT problem. Thus the latter is strongly NP-hard due to Theorem 5.

The most versatile approach to deal with the TT problem including different kinds of constraints, is by integer programming as done by [25]. They first formulate the decomposition time problem as an integer linear program (IP), where interleaf motion, width, or tongue-and-groove constraints can easily be written as linear constraints. The optimal objective $z = DT(\alpha)$ can then be used in a modified IP as upper bound for the decomposition time which is now treated as variable (rather than objective) and in which the number of C1 matrices is to be minimized. This approach can be considered as an ε-constraint method to solve bicriteria optimization problems (see, for instance, [16]). The solutions in [25] can thus be interpreted as Pareto optimal solutions with respect to the two objective functions $DT(\alpha)$ and $DC(\alpha)$. Due to the large number of variables, the algorithm presented in [25] is, however, not usable for realistic problem instances.

The importance of conflict between the DT and DC objectives has not been investigated to a great extent. The author in [3] showed that for matrices with a single row there is always a decomposition that minimizes both $DC(\alpha)$ and $DT(\alpha)$. The following examples show that the optimal solutions of the (unconstrained) DT, DC and TT_{var} problems are in general attained in different decompositions. As a consequence, it is not enough to find the best possible decomposition cardinality among all decompositions with minimal decomposition time as is done in most papers on the DC problem (see Section 3). We will present next an example which is the smallest possible one for different optimal solutions of the DT and DC problems.

Example 1. Let

$$A = \begin{pmatrix} 3 & 6 & 4 \\ 2 & 1 & 5 \end{pmatrix}.$$

Since the entries $1, \dots, 6$ can only be uniquely represented by the numbers $1, 2$ and 4, the unique optimal decomposition of the DC problem is given by $A = 1Y^1 + 2Y^2 + 4Y^3$ where

$$Y^1 = \begin{pmatrix} 1 & 0 & 0 \\ 0 & 1 & 1 \end{pmatrix}, Y^2 = \begin{pmatrix} 1 & 1 & 0 \\ 1 & 0 & 0 \end{pmatrix}, \quad \text{and} \quad Y^3 = \begin{pmatrix} 0 & 1 & 1 \\ 0 & 0 & 1 \end{pmatrix}.$$

Hence, the optimal value of the DC problem is 3, with $DT = 7$. Since the optimal solution of the DT problem has $DT = 6$, we conclude that $DC \geq 4$.

It is not clear whether this example is of practical value. In Section 5 we see that in our tests the optimal solution of the DC problem examples was not among the DT optimal solutions in only 5 out of 32 examples. In these cases the difference in the DC objective was only 1. This is also emphasized by [26] who confirm that the conflict between DT and DC is often small in practice.

Another possible combination of objective functions is the treatment time problem with variable set-up time $TT_{var}(\alpha) := DT(\alpha) + SU_{var}(\alpha) = DT(\alpha) + \sum_{k=1}^{K-1} \tau_{\pi(k),\pi(k+1)}$ (see (6)). Minimizing $TT_{var}(\alpha)$ is strongly NP-hard when looking at the special case $\tau_{kl} = \tau$ for all k, l, which yields the objective function of $TT_{const}(\alpha)$. Here, we consider

$$\tau_{\pi(k),\pi(k+1)} = \max_{m \in \mathcal{M}} \max \left\{ |l_m^{\pi(k)} - l_m^{\pi(k+1)}|, |r_m^{\pi(k)} - r_m^{\pi(k+1)}| \right\}, \qquad (14)$$

i.e., the maximal number of positions any leave moves between two consecutive matrices $Y^{\pi(k)}$ and $Y^{\pi(k+1)}$ in the sequence.

Extending Example 1, the following example shows that the three objective functions $DT(\alpha)$, $DC(\alpha)$, and $TT_{var}(\alpha)$ yield, in general, different optimal solutions.

Example 2. Let

$$A = \begin{pmatrix} 8 & 5 & 6 \\ 5 & 3 & 6 \end{pmatrix}.$$

The optimal decomposition for DC is

$$A = 5 \begin{pmatrix} 1 & 1 & 0 \\ 1 & 0 & 0 \end{pmatrix} + 3 \begin{pmatrix} 1 & 0 & 0 \\ 0 & 1 & 0 \end{pmatrix} + 6 \begin{pmatrix} 0 & 0 & 1 \\ 0 & 0 & 1 \end{pmatrix}.$$

This decomposition yields $DT = 14$, $DC = 3$ and $TT_{var} = DT + SU_{var} = 14 + 3 = 17$, where $SU_{var} = 1 + 2 = 3$. The optimal decomposition for DT is

$$A = 3 \begin{pmatrix} 1 & 0 & 0 \\ 0 & 0 & 1 \end{pmatrix} + \begin{pmatrix} 0 & 0 & 1 \\ 0 & 1 & 1 \end{pmatrix} + 3 \begin{pmatrix} 1 & 1 & 1 \\ 1 & 0 & 0 \end{pmatrix} + 2 \begin{pmatrix} 1 & 1 & 1 \\ 1 & 1 & 1 \end{pmatrix}.$$

Here we obtain $DT = 9$, $DC = 4$, $SU_{var} = 2 + 2 + 2 = 6$ and thus $TT_{var} = 15$. The optimal decomposition for TT_{var} is

$$A = 2 \begin{pmatrix} 0 & 0 & 1 \\ 1 & 1 & 1 \end{pmatrix} + 3 \begin{pmatrix} 1 & 0 & 0 \\ 1 & 0 & 0 \end{pmatrix} + \begin{pmatrix} 1 & 1 & 0 \\ 0 & 1 & 0 \end{pmatrix} + 4 \begin{pmatrix} 1 & 1 & 1 \\ 0 & 0 & 1 \end{pmatrix}.$$

We get $DT = 10$, $DC = 4$ and $SU_{var} = 2 + 1 + 1 = 4$, leading to $TT_{var} = 14$.

If the set of C1 matrices $Y^1, \ldots, Y^K$ in the formulation $TT_{var}(\alpha)$ is given, one can apply a traveling salesman algorithm to minimize $SU_{var}(\alpha)$. Since the number L of C1 matrices is in general rather small, the TSP can be solved exactly in reasonable time. If the set of C1 matrices is not given, the problem becomes a simultaneous decomposition and sequencing problem which is currently under research.

5 Numerical results

Very few numerical comparisons are available in the literature. The author in [29] compares in his numerical investigations eight different heuristics for the DC problem. He concludes that the Algorithm of Xia and Verhey [33] outperforms its competitors. With new algorithms developed since the appearance of Que's paper, the dominance of the Xia-Verhey algorithm is no longer true, as observed by [15] and seen below.

In this section we present results obtained with the majority of algorithms mentioned in this paper for constrained and unconstrained problems. We consider only interleaf motion constraints, since these are the most common and incorporated in most algorithms. As seen in Section 2 the unconstrained and constrained DT problems can be solved in $\mathcal{O}(NM)$, respectively $\mathcal{O}(NM^2)$ time. Moreover, we found that algorithms that guarantee minimal $DT(\alpha)$ and include a heuristic to reduce $DC(\alpha)$ do not require significantly higher CPU time. Therefore we exclude algorithms that simply minimize $DT(\alpha)$ without control over $DC(\alpha)$. Table 1 shows the references for the algorithms, and some remarks on their properties.

We used 47 clinical examples varying in size from 5 to 23 rows and 6 to 30 columns, with L varying between 9 and 40. In addition, we used 15 instances of size 10×10 with entries randomly generated between 1 and 14. In all experiments we have applied an (exact) TSP algorithm to the resulting matrices to minimize the total treatment time for the given decomposition. Table 2 presents the results for the unconstrained and Table 3 presents those for the constrained problems. All experiments were run on a Pentium 4 PC with 2.4 GHz and 512 MB RAM. In both tables we first show the number of instances for which the algorithms gave the best values for DT, DC and TT_{var} after application of the TSP to the matrices produced by the algorithms. Next, we list the maximal CPU time (in seconds) the algorithm took for any of the instances. The next four rows show the minimum, maximum, median, and average relative deviation from the best DC value found by any of the algorithms. The next four rows show the same for TT_{var}. Finally, we list the improvement of variable setup time according to (14) obtained by applying the TSP to the matrices found by the algorithms.

Table 1. List of algorithms tested.

Algorithm	Problem	Remarks
Baatar et al. [5]	unconstrained	guarantees min DT, heuristic for DC
Engel [18]	unconstrained	guarantees min DT, heuristic for DC
Xia and Verhey [33]	unconstrained	heuristic for DC
Baatar et al. [5]	constrained	guarantees min DT, heuristic for DC
Kalinowski [22]	constrained	guarantees min DT, heuristic for DC
Siochi [32]	constrained	guarantees min DT, heuristic for TT
Xia and Verhey [33]	constrained	heuristic for DC

Table 2. Numerical results for the unconstrained algorithms.

		Baatar et al. [5]	Engel [18]	Xia and Verhey [33]
Best DT		62	62	0
Best DC		7	62	1
Best TT_{var}		38	17	9
Best CPU		0	21	45
Max CPU		0.1157	0.0820	0.0344
$\Delta\,DC$	Min	0.00%	0.00%	0.00%
	Max	33.33%	0.00%	86.67%
	Median	18.18%	0.00%	36.93%
	Mean	17.08%	0.00%	37.82%
$\Delta\,TT$	Min	0.00%	0.00%	0.00%
	Max	21.30%	42.38%	83.82%
	Median	0.00%	5.66%	14.51%
	Mean	3.14%	8.74%	17.23%
$\Delta\,SU$	Min	0.83%	1.43%	7.89%
	Max	37.50%	27.27%	43.40%
	Median	14.01%	10.46%	25.41%
	Mean	13.91%	12.15%	25.74%

Table 3. Numerical results for the constrained algorithms.

		Baatar et al. [5]	Kalinowski [22]	Siochi [32]	Xia and Verhey [33]
Best DT		62	62	62	0
Best DC		1	62	1	0
Best TT_{var}		12	43	11	0
Best CPU		0	0	0	62
Max CPU		0.2828	0.8071	1.4188	0.0539
$\Delta\,DC$	Min	0.00%	0.00%	0.00%	11.11%
	Max	160.00%	0.00%	191.67%	355.56%
	Median	70.71%	0.00%	108.12%	70.71%
	Mean	71.37%	0.00%	102.39%	86.58%
$\Delta\,TT$	Min	0.00%	0.00%	0.00%	10.66%
	Max	50.74%	45.28%	26.47%	226.42%
	Median	5.23%	0.00%	8.49%	51.03%
	Mean	7.97%	4.95%	8.26%	61.56%
$\Delta\,SU$	Min	0.00%	2.27%	0.00%	5.00%
	Max	18.18%	35.25%	20.00%	24.05%
	Median	4.45%	22.45%	2.11%	14.20%
	Mean	5.34%	21.66%	3.24%	14.42%

Table 4. Comparison of Kalinowski [21] and Nußbaum [28]. A * next to the DC value indicates a difference between the algorithms.

Data Sets	Kalinowski [21]				Nußbaum [28]			
	DT	DC	TT	CPU	DT	DC	TT	CPU
Clinical 1	27	7	49	0	27	7	49	0
Clinical 2	27	6	43	1	27	6	43	1
Clinical 3	24	8	59	2	28	7*	56	213
Clinical 4	33	6	48	1	33	6	48	1
Clinical 5	41	9	76	41	44	8*	73	134
Clinical 6	13	8	125	8	13	8	125	8
Clinical 7	12	9	134	27	12	9	134	27
Clinical 8	12	8	153	15	12	8	153	15
Clinical 9	12	9	118	174	12	9	118	174
Clinical 10	11	9	108	133	11	9	108	133
Clinical 11	11	6	97	0	11	6	97	0
Clinical 12	10	7	99	0	10	7	99	0
Clinical 14	17	8	48	0	17	8	48	0
Clinical 15	19	7	54	0	19	7	54	0
Clinical 16	15	7	46	0	15	7	46	0
Clinical 17	16	7	48	0	16	7	48	0
Clinical 18	20	8	50	4	20	8	50	9
Clinical 19	16	7	51	0	16	7	51	0
Clinical 20	18	7	47	0	18	7	47	0
Clinical 21	22	8	65	1	22	8	65	1
Clinical 22	22	10	74	10	25	9*	81	23
Clinical 23	26	9	76	24	26	9	76	24
Clinical 24	23	9	63	6	23	9	63	7
Clinical 25	23	9	75	12	23	9	75	13
Clinical 26	22	9	68	2	22	9	68	2
Clinical 39	28	10	88	149	28	10	88	149
Clinical 40	26	8	60	2	27	7*	55	3
Clinical 41	20	7	46	1	20	7	46	1
Clinical 42	23	8	55	0	23	8	55	0
Clinical 45	21	6	42	0	21	6	42	0
Clinical 46	19	9	65	10	21	8*	59	40
Clinical 47	24	10	85	1	24	10	85	1

Table 2 shows that Xia and Verhey [33] is the fastest algorithm. However, it never found the optimal DT value and found the best DC value for only one instance. Since the largest CPU time is 0.116 seconds, computation time is not an issue. Thus we conclude that Xia and Verhey [33] is inferior to the other algorithms. Baatar et al. [5] and Engel [18] are roughly equal in speed. Both guarantee optimal DT, but the latter performs better in terms of DC, finding the best value for all instances. However, the slightly greater amount of matrices used by the former method appears to enable better TT_{var} values and a slightly bigger improvement of the variable setup time by reordering the segments. We observe that applying a TSP algorithm is clearly worthwhile, reducing the variable setup time by up to 40%.

The results for the constrained problems underline that the algorithm of [33], despite being the fastest for all instances, is not competitive. It did not find the best DT, DC, or TT_{var} values for any example. The other three algorithms guarantee DT optimality. The algorithm of [22] performs best, finding the best DC value in all cases, and the best TT_{var} value in 43 of the 62 tests. Baatar et al. [5] and Siochi [32] are comparable, with the former being slightly better in terms of DC, TT_{var} and CPU time. Again, the application of a TSP algorithm is well worth the effort to reduce the variable setup time.

Finally, the results of comparing the algorithm of [21] with its new iterative version of [28] on a subset of the clinical instances are given in Table 4. These tests were performed on a PC with Dual Xeon Processor, 3.2 GHz and 4 GB RAM. In the comparison of 32 clinical cases there were only five cases (3, 5, 22, 40, 46) where the optimal solution of the DC problem was not among the optimal solutions of the DT problem — and thus found by the algorithm of [21]. In these five cases, the DC objective was only reduced by a value of 1. Since the iterative algorithm performs at most $NML - DT$ applications of Kalinowski-like procedures, the CPU time is obviously considerably larger.

Acknowledgements

The authors thank David Craigie, Zhenzhen Mu, and Dong Zhang, who implemented most of the algorithms, and Thomas Kalinowski for providing the source code of his algorithms.

References

1. R. K. Ahuja and H. W. Hamacher. A network flow algorithm to minimize beam-on-time for unconstrained multileaf collimator problems in cancer radiation therapy. *Networks*, 45:36–41, 2004.
2. R. K. Ahuja, T. L. Magnanti, and J. B. Orlin. *Network Flows: Theory, Algorithms and Applications*. Prentice-Hall, 1993.
3. D. Baatar. *Matrix Decomposition with Time and Cardinality Objectives: Theory, Algorithms, and Application to Multileaf Collimator Sequencing*. PhD thesis, Department of Mathematics, Technical University of Kaiserslautern, 2005.
4. D. Baatar and H. W. Hamacher. New LP model for multileaf collimators in radiation therapy planning. In *Proceedings of the Operations Research Peripatetic Postgraduate Programme Conference ORP³, Lambrecht, Germany*, pages 11–29, 2003.
5. D. Baatar, H. W. Hamacher, M. Ehrgott, and G. J. Woeginger. Decomposition of integer matrices and multileaf collimator sequencing. *Discrete Applied Mathematics*, 152:6–34, 2005.

6. Nikhil Bansal, Don Coppersmith, and Baruch Schieber. Minimizing setup and beam-on times in radiation therapy. In Josep Díaz, Klaus Jansen, José D. P. Rolim, and Uri Zwick, editors, *APPROX-RANDOM. Approximation, Randomization, and Combinatorial Optimization. Algorithms and Techniques, 9th International Workshop on Approximation Algorithms for Combinatorial Optimization Problems, APPROX 2006 and 10th International Workshop on Randomization and Computation, RANDOM 2006, Barcelona, Spain, August 28-30 2006, Proceedings*, volume 4110 of *Lecture Notes in Computer Science*, pages 27–38. Springer Verlag, Berlin, 2006.

7. N. Boland, H. W. Hamacher, and F. Lenzen. Minimizing beam-on-time in cancer radiation treatment using multileaf collimators. *Networks*, 43:226–240, 2004.

8. T. R. Bortfeld, A. L. Boyer, D. L. Kahler, and T. J. Waldron. X-ray field compensation with multileaf collimators. *International Journal of Radiation Oncology, Biology, Physics*, 28:723–730, 1994.

9. R. E. Burkard. Open Problem Session, Oberwolfach Conference on Combinatorial Optimization, November 24–29, 2002.

10. D. Z. Chen, X. S. Hu, S. Luan, C. Wang, S. A. Naqvi, and C. X. Yu. Generalized geometric approaches for leaf sequencing problems in radiation therapy. In *Proceedings of the 15th Annual International Symposium on Algorithms and Computation (ISAAC), Hong Kong, December 2004*, volume 3341 of *Lecture Notes in Computer Science*, pages 271–281. Springer Verlag, Berlin, 2004.

11. D. Z. Chen, X. S. Hu, S. Luan, C. Wang, S. A. Naqvi, and C. X. Yu. Generalized geometric approaches for leaf sequencing problems in radiation therapy. *International Journal of Computational Geometry and Applications*, 16(2-3):175–204, 2006.

12. D. Z. Chen, X. S. Hu, S. Luan, C. Wang, and X. Wu. Geometric algorithms for static leaf sequencing problems in radiation therapy. *International Journal of Computational Geometry and Applications*, 14:311–339, 2004.

13. D. Z. Chen, X. S. Hu, S. Luan, X. Wu, and C. X. Yu. Optimal terrain construction problems and applications in intensity-modulated radiation therapy. *Algorithmica*, 42:265–288, 2005.

14. M. J. Collins, D. Kempe, J. Saia, and M. Young. Nonnegative integral subset representations of integer sets. *Information Processing Letters*, 101:129–133, 2007.

15. S. M. Crooks, L. F. McAven, D. F. Robinson, and L. Xing. Minimizing delivery time and monitor units in static IMRT by leaf-sequencing. *Physics in Medicine and Biology*, 47:3105–3116, 2002.

16. M. Ehrgott. *Multicriteria Optimization*. Springer Verlag, Berlin, 2nd edition, 2005.

17. M. Ehrgott, A. Holder, and J. Reese. Beam selection in radiotherapy design. *Linear Algebra and its Applications*, doi: 10.1016/j.laa.2007.05.039, 2007.

18. K. Engel. A new algorithm for optimal MLC field segmentation. *Discrete Applied Mathematics*, 152:35–51, 2005.

19. A. D. A. Gunawardena, W. D'Souza, L. D. Goadrick, R. R. Meyer, K. J. Sorensen, S. A. Naqvi, and L. Shi. A difference-matrix metaheuristic for intensity map segmentation in step-and-shoot imrt delivery. *Physics in Medicine and Biology*, 51:2517–2536, 2006.

20. H. W. Hamacher and K.-H. Küfer. Inverse radiation therapy planing – A multiple objective optimization approach. *Discrete Applied Mathematics*, 118:145–161, 2002.

21. T. Kalinowski. Algorithmic complexity of the minimization of the number of segments in multileaf collimator field segmentation. Technical report, Department of Mathematics, University of Rostock, 2004. Preprint 2004/1.

22. T. Kalinowski. A duality based algorithm for multileaf collimator field segmentation with interleaf collision constraint. *Discrete Applied Mathematics*, 152:52–88, 2005.

23. S. Kamath, S. Sahni, J. Li, J. Palta, and S. Ranka. Leaf sequencing algorithms for segmented multileaf collimation. *Physics in Medicine and Biology*, 48:307–324, 2003.

24. S. Kamath, S. Sahni, S. Ranka, J. Li, and J. Palta. A comparison of step-and-shoot leaf sequencing algorithms that eliminate tongue-and-groove effects. *Physics in Medicine and Biology*, 49:3137–3143, 2004.

25. M. Langer, V. Thai, and L. Papiez. Improved leaf sequencing reduces segments of monitor units needed to deliver IMRT using MLC. *Medical Physics*, 28:2450–58, 2001.

26. M. P. Langer, V. Thai, and L. Papiez. Tradeoffs between segments and monitor units are not required for static field IMRT delivery. *International Journal of Radiation Oncology, Biology, Physics*, 51:75, 2001.

27. S. Luan, J. Saia, and M. Young. Approximation algorithms for minimizing segments in radiation therapy. *Information Processin Letters*, 101:239–244, 2007.

28. M. Nußbaum. Min cardinality c1-decomposition of integer matrices. Master's thesis, Department of Mathematics, Technical University of Kaiserslautern, 2006.

29. W. Que. Comparison of algorithms for multileaf collimator field segmentation. *Medical Physics*, 26:2390–2396, 1999.

30. L. Shao. A survey of beam intensity optimization in imrt. In T. Halliburton, editor, *Proceedings of the 40th Annual Conference of the Operational Research Society of New Zealand, Wellington, 2-3 December 2005*, pages 255–264, 2005. Available online at **http://secure.orsnz.org.nz/conf40/content/paper/Shao.pdf**.

31. D. M. Shepard, M. C. Ferris, G. H. Olivera, and T. R. Mackie. Optimizing the delivery of radiation therapy to cancer patients. *SIAM Review*, 41:721–744, 1999.

32. R. A. C. Siochi. Minimizing static intensity modulation delivery time using an intensity solid paradigm. *International Journal of Radiation Oncology, Biology, Physics*, 43:671–689, 1999.

33. P. Xia and L. Verhey. Multileaf collimator leaf sequencing algorithm for intensity modulated beams with multiple segments. *Medical Physics*, 25:1424–1434, 1998.

Appendix: The instances

Tables 5 and 6 show the size (N, M, L) of the instances, the optimal value of $DT(\alpha)$ in the constrained and unconstrained problems, and the best $DC(\alpha)$ and $TT_{var}(\alpha)$ values found by any of the tested algorithms, with a * indicating proven optimality for DC in the unconstrained case.

Table 5. The 15 random instances.

Data Set	Size			Unconstrained			Constrained		
	M	N	L	DT	DC	TT	DT	DC	TT
Random 1	10	10	14	37	11	107	39	16	110
Random 2	10	10	14	30	11	102	33	13	100
Random 3	10	10	14	36	11	103	37	16	106
Random 4	10	10	14	37	11	114	37	12	99
Random 5	10	10	14	46	12	120	46	16	107
Random 6	10	10	14	45	12	123	45	14	112
Random 7	10	10	14	41	11	117	47	16	122
Random 8	10	10	14	41	12	119	41	15	106
Random 9	10	10	14	33	11	102	33	13	98
Random 10	10	10	14	34	10	94	40	15	102
Random 11	10	10	14	41	11	113	41	14	102
Random 12	10	10	14	35	11	106	37	15	102
Random 13	10	10	14	32	11	105	32	13	99
Random 14	10	10	14	43	11	114	43	18	112
Random 15	10	10	14	36	10	109	37	14	107

Table 6. The 47 clinical instances.

Data Set	Size			Unconstrained			Constrained		
	M	N	L	DT	DC	TT	DT	DC	TT
Clinical 1	5	6	23	27	7*	49	27	8	51
Clinical 2	5	7	27	27	6*	43	27	8	48
Clinical 3	5	8	18	24	7*	54	24	8	53
Clinical 4	5	7	30	33	6*	48	33	8	51
Clinical 5	5	8	25	41	8*	73	41	10	73
Clinical 6	16	29	10	13	8*	125	13	9	132
Clinical 7	16	27	10	12	9*	122	12	9	138
Clinical 8	16	30	10	12	8*	135	15	11	163
Clinical 9	15	28	9	12	9*	118	12	9	151
Clinical 10	16	28	10	11	9*	108	11	10	106
Clinical 11	20	23	10	11	6*	96	11	7	136
Clinical 12	16	28	10	10	7*	99	13	10	130
Clinical 13	20	25	9	17	11	151	17	12	130
Clinical 14	9	9	10	17	8*	38	17	9	50
Clinical 15	9	10	10	19	7*	53	19	11	62
Clinical 16	10	9	10	15	7*	44	18	9	50
Clinical 17	10	9	10	16	7*	45	16	8	47
Clinical 18	9	9	10	20	8*	50	20	10	49
Clinical 19	10	10	10	16	7*	50	16	8	57
Clinical 20	10	9	10	18	7*	47	18	9	56

(continued)

Table 6. Continued.

Data Set	Size			Unconstrained			Constrained		
	M	N	L	DT	DC	TT	DT	DC	TT
Clinical 21	14	10	10	22	8*	65	23	13	73
Clinical 22	14	10	10	22	9*	74	22	11	79
Clinical 23	14	10	10	26	9*	76	30	15	89
Clinical 24	14	10	10	23	9*	63	24	11	79
Clinical 25	14	10	10	23	9*	74	23	12	84
Clinical 26	14	10	10	22	9*	68	22	10	70
Clinical 27	22	23	24	33	14	165	34	17	158
Clinical 28	23	17	27	46	15	184	46	17	186
Clinical 29	23	16	33	35	12	155	48	17	174
Clinical 30	22	21	31	50	15	197	58	21	196
Clinical 31	22	22	22	47	15	205	58	21	201
Clinical 32	22	15	26	33	11	134	42	16	142
Clinical 33	22	18	24	41	13	186	41	18	175
Clinical 34	9	13	29	45	13	147	45	15	129
Clinical 35	9	10	40	59	11	103	69	14	124
Clinical 36	9	12	26	45	12	131	45	14	111
Clinical 37	9	10	35	46	11	115	46	12	116
Clinical 38	11	11	19	35	9	68	35	10	79
Clinical 39	11	11	22	28	10*	84	33	14	91
Clinical 40	11	12	19	26	7*	55	27	10	75
Clinical 41	11	9	16	20	7*	46	22	8	52
Clinical 42	11	9	14	23	8*	55	23	10	58
Clinical 43	11	12	26	43	11	101	49	16	119
Clinical 44	10	15	26	49	13	137	54	16	114
Clinical 45	11	8	21	21	6*	48	21	9	49
Clinical 46	11	12	16	19	8*	42	19	10	66
Clinical 47	11	14	22	24	10*	59	38	15	105

Neuro-dynamic programming for fractionated radiotherapy planning*

Geng Deng[1] and Michael C. Ferris[2]

[1] Department of Mathematics, University of Wisconsin at Madison, 480 Lincoln Dr., Madison, WI 53706, USA, geng@cs.wisc.edu
[2] Computer Sciences Department, University of Wisconsin at Madison, 1210 W. Dayton Street, Madison, WI 53706, USA, ferris@cs.wisc.edu

Summary. We investigate an on-line planning strategy for the fractionated radiotherapy planning problem, which incorporates the effects of day-to-day patient motion. On-line planning demonstrates significant improvement over off-line strategies in terms of reducing registration error, but it requires extra work in the replanning procedures, such as in the CT scans and the re-computation of a deliverable dose profile. We formulate the problem in a dynamic programming framework and solve it based on the approximate policy iteration techniques of neuro-dynamic programming. In initial limited testing, the solutions we obtain outperform existing solutions and offer an improved dose profile for each fraction of the treatment.

Keywords: Fractionation, adaptive radiation therapy, neuro-dynamic programming, reinforcement learning.

1 Introduction

Every year, nearly 500,000 patients in the United States are treated with external beam radiation, the most common form of radiation therapy. Before receiving irradiation, the patient is imaged using computed tomography (CT) or magnetic resonance imaging (MRI). The physician contours the tumor and surrounding critical structures on these images and prescribes a dose of radiation to be delivered to the tumor. *Intensity-Modulated Radiotherapy* (IMRT) is one of the most powerful tools to deliver conformal dose to a tumor target [6, 17, 23]. The treatment process involves optimization over specific parameters, such as angle selection and (pencil) beam weights [8, 9, 16, 18]. The organs near the tumor will inevitably receive radiation as well; the

* This material is based on research partially supported by the National Science Foundation Grants DMS-0427689 and IIS-0511905 and the Air Force Office of Scientific Research Grant FA9550-04-1-0192.

physician places constraints on how much radiation each organ should receive. The dose is then delivered by radiotherapy devices, typically in a fractionated regime consisting of five doses per week for a period of 4-9 weeks [10].

Generally, the use of fractionation is known to increase the probability of controlling the tumor and to decrease damage to normal tissue surrounding the tumor. However, the motion of the patient or the internal organs between treatment sessions can result in failure to deliver adequate radiation to the tumor [14, 21]. We classify the delivery error in the following types:

1. *Registration Error* (see Figure 1 (a)). Registration error is due to the incorrect positioning of the patient in day-to-day treatment. This is the *interfraction error* we primarily consider in this paper. Accuracy in patient positioning during treatment set-up is a requirement for precise delivery. Traditional positioning techniques include laser alignment to skin markers. Such methods are highly prone to error and in general show a

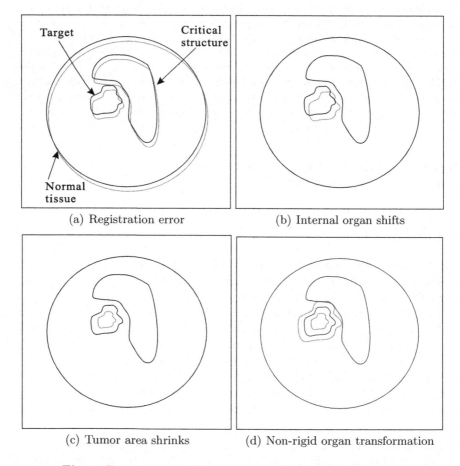

(a) Registration error   (b) Internal organ shifts

(c) Tumor area shrinks   (d) Non-rigid organ transformation

Fig. 1. Four types of delivery error in hypo-fraction treatment.

displacement variation of 4-7mm depending on the site treated. Other advanced devices, such as electronic portal imaging systems, can reduce the registration error by comparing real-time digital images to facilitate a time-efficient patient repositioning [17].

2. *Internal Organ Motion Error*, (Figure 1 (b)). The error is caused by the internal motion of organs and tissues in a human body. For example, intracranial tissue shifts up to 1.5 mm when patients change position from prone to supine. The use of implanted radio-opaque markers allows physicians to verify the displacement of organs.

3. *Tumor Shrinkage Error*, (Figure 1 (c)). This error is due to tumor area shrinkage as the treatment progresses. The originally prescribed dose delivered to target tissue does not reflect the change in tumor area. For example, the tumor can shrink up to 30% in volume within three treatments.

4. *Non-rigid Transformation Error*, (Figure 1 (d)). This type of intrafraction motion error is internally induced by non-rigid deformation of organs, including for example, lung and cardiac motion in normal breathing conditions.

In our model formulation, we consider only the registration error between fractions and neglect the other three types of error. Internal organ motion error occurs during delivery and is therefore categorized as an *intrafraction error*. Our methods are not real-time solution techniques at this stage and consequently are not applicable to this setting. Tumor shrinkage error and non-rigid transformation error mainly occur between treatment sessions and are therefore called interfraction errors. However, the changes in the tumor in these cases are not volume preserving, and incorporating such effects remains a topic of future research. The principal computational difficulty arises in that setting from the mapping of voxels between two stages.

Off-line planning is currently widespread. It only involves a single planning step and delivers the same amount of dose at each stage. It was suggested in [5, 15, 19] that an optimal inverse plan should incorporate an estimated probability distribution of the patient motion during the treatment. Such distribution of patient geometry can be estimated [7, 12], for example, using a few pre-scanned images, by techniques such as Bayesian inference [20]. The probability distributions vary among organs and patients.

An alternative delivery scheme is so called on-line planning, which includes multiple planning steps during the treatment. Each planning step uses feedback from images generated during treatment, for example, by CT scans. On-line replanning accurately captures the changing requirements for radiation dose at each stage, but it inevitably consumes much more time during every replanning procedure.

This paper aims at formulating a *dynamic programming* (DP) framework that solves the day-to-day on-line planning problem. The optimal policy is selected from several candidate deliverable dose profiles, compensating over time for movement of the patient. The techniques are based on neuro-dynamic programming (NDP) ideas [3]. In the next section, we introduce the model formulation and in Section 3, we describe serval types of approximation architecture and the NDP methods we employ. We give computational results on a real patient case in Section 4.

2 Model formulation

To describe the problem more precisely, suppose the treatment lasts N periods (stages), and the state $x_k(i), k = 0, 1, \ldots, N, i \in \mathcal{T}$, contains the actual dose delivered to all voxels after k stages (x_k is obtained through a replanning process). Here $\mathcal{T}$ represents the collection of voxels in the target organ. The state evolves as a discrete-time dynamic system:

$$x_{k+1} = \phi(x_k, u_k, \omega_k), \ k = 0, 1, \ldots, N - 1, \tag{1}$$

where u_k is the control (namely dose applied) at the kth stage, and ω_k is a (typically three dimensional) random vector representing the uncertainty of patient positioning. Normally, we assume that ω_k corresponds to a shift transformation to u_k. Hence the function ϕ has the explicit form

$$\phi(x_k(i), u_k(i), \omega_k) = x_k(i) + u_k(i + \omega_k), \ \forall i \in \mathcal{T}. \tag{2}$$

Since each treatment is delivered separately and in succession, we also assume the uncertainty vector ω_k is i.i.d. In the context of voxelwise shifts, ω_k is regarded as a discretely distributed random vector. The control u_k is drawn from an applicable control set $U(x_k)$.

Since there is no recourse for dose delivered outside of the target, an instantaneous error (or cost) $g(x_k, x_{k+1}, u_k)$ is incurred when evolving between stage x_k and x_{k+1}. Let the final state x_N represent the total dose delivered on the target during the treatment period. At the end of N stages, a terminal cost $J_N(x_N)$ will be evaluated. Thus, the plan chooses controls $\boldsymbol{u} = \{u_0, u_1, \ldots, u_{N-1}\}$ so as to minimize an expected total cost:

$$J_0(x_0) = \min \mathbb{E} \left[\sum_{k=0}^{N-1} g(x_k, x_{k+1}, u_k) + J_N(x_N) \right]$$
$$s.t. \ x_{k+1} = \phi(x_k, u_k, \omega_k), \tag{3}$$
$$u_k \in U(x_k), k = 0, 1, \ldots, N - 1.$$

We use the notation $J_0(x_0)$ to represent an optimal cost-to-go function that accumulates the expected optimal cost starting at stage 0 with the initial state x_0. Moreover, if we extend the definition to a general stage, the cost-to-go function J_j defined at j^{th} stage is expressed in a recursive pattern,

$$J_j(x_j)$$

$$= \min \mathbb{E} \left[\sum_{k=j}^{N-1} g(x_k, x_{k+1}, u_k) + J_N(x_N) \, \middle| \, \begin{array}{l} x_{k+1} = \phi(x_k, u_k, \omega_k), \\ u_k \in U(x_k), k = j, \ldots, N-1 \end{array} \right]$$

$$= \min \mathbb{E} \left[g(x_j, x_{j+1}, u_j) + J_{j+1}(x_{j+1}) \mid x_{j+1} = \phi(x_j, u_j, \omega_j), u_j \in U(x_j) \right].$$

For ease of exposition, we assume that the final cost function is a linear combination of the absolute differences between the current dose and the ideal target dose at each voxel. That is

$$J_N(x_N) = \sum_{i \in T} p(i)|x_N(i) - T(i)|. \tag{4}$$

Here, $T(i), i \in T$ in voxel i represents the required final dosage on the target, and the vector p weights the importance of hitting the ideal value for each voxel. We typically set $p(i) = 10$, for $i \in T$, and $p(i) = 1$ elsewhere, in our problem to emphasize the importance of target volume. Other forms of final cost function could be used, such as the sum of least squares error [19].

A key issue to note is that the controls are nonnegative since dose cannot be removed from the patient. The immediate cost g at each stage is the amount of dose delivered outside of the target volume due to the random shift,

$$g(x_k, x_{k+1}, u_k) = \sum_{i+\omega_k \notin T} p(i + \omega_k) u_k(i + \omega_k). \tag{5}$$

It is clear that the immediate cost is only associated with the control u_k and the random term ω_k. If there is no displacement error ($\omega_k = 0$), the immediate cost is 0, corresponding to the case of accurate delivery.

The control most commonly used in the clinic is the constant policy, which delivers

$$u_k = T/N$$

at each stage and ignores the errors and uncertainties. (As mentioned in the introduction, when the planner knows the probability distribution, an optimal off-line planning strategy calculates a total dose profile D, which is later divided by N and delivered using the constant policy, so that the expected delivery after N stages is close to T.) We propose an on-line planning strategy that attempts to compensate for the error over the remaining time stages. At each time stage, we divide the residual dose required by the remaining time stages:

$$u_k = \max(0, T - x_k)/(N - k).$$

Since the reactive policy takes into consideration the residual at each time stage, we expect this reactive policy to outperform the constant policy. Note the reactive policy requires knowledge of the cumulative dose x_k and replanning at every stage — a significant additional computation burden over current practice.

We illustrate later in this paper how the constant and reactive heuristic policies perform on several examples. We also explain how the NDP approach improves upon these results. The NDP makes decisions on several candidate policies (so-called modified reactive policies), which account for a variation of intensities on the reactive policy. At each stage, given an amplifying parameter a on the overall intensity level, the policy delivers

$$u_k = a \cdot \max(0, T - x_k)/(N - k).$$

We will show that the amplifying range of $a > 1$ is preferable to $a = 1$, which is equivalent to the standard reactive policy. The parameter a should be confined with an upper bound, so that the total delivery does not exceed the tolerance level of normal tissue.

Note that we assume these idealized policies u_k (the constant, reactive and modified reactive policies) are valid and deliverable in our model. However, in practice they are not because u_k has to be a combination of dose profiles of beamlets fired from a gantry. In Voelker's thesis [22], some techniques to approximate u_k are provided. Furthermore, as delivering devices and planning tools become more sophisticated, such policies will become attainable.

So far, the fractionation problem is formulated in a *finite horizon*[3] dynamic programming framework [1, 4, 13]. Numerous techniques for such problems can be applied to compute optimal decision policies. But unfortunately, because of the immensity of these state spaces (Bellman's "curse of dimensionality"), the classical dynamic programming algorithm is inapplicable. For instance, in a simple one-dimensional problem with only ten voxels involving 6 time stages, the DP solution times are around one-half hour. To address these complex problems, we design sub-optimal solutions using approximate DP algorithms — *neuro-dynamic programming* [3, 11].

3 Neuro-dynamic programming

3.1 Introduction

Neuro-dynamic programming is a class of reinforcement learning methods that approximate the optimal cost-to-go function. Bertsekas and Tsitsiklis [3] coined the term neuro-dynamic programming because it is associated with building and tuning a neural network via simulation results. The idea of an approximate cost function helps NDP avoid the curse of dimensionality and distinguishes the NDP methods from earlier approximation versions of DP methods. Sub-optimal DP solutions are obtained at significantly smaller computational costs.

The central issue we consider is the evaluation and approximation of the reduced optimal cost function J_k in the setting of the radiation fractionation

---

[3] Finite horizon means finite number of stages.

problem — a finite horizon problem with N periods. We will approximate a total of N optimal cost-to-go functions $J_k, k = 0, 1, \ldots, N - 1$, by simulation and training of a neural network. We replace the optimal cost $J_k(\cdot)$ with an approximate function $\tilde{J}_k(\cdot, r_k)$ (all of the $\tilde{J}_k(\cdot, r_k)$ have the same parametric form), where r_k is a vector of parameters to be ascertained from a training process. The function $\tilde{J}_k(\cdot, r_k)$ is called a scoring function, and the value $\tilde{J}_k(x, r_k)$ is called the score of state x. We use the optimal control $\hat{u}_k$ that solves the minimum problem in the (approximation of the) right-hand-side of Bellman's equation defined using

$$\hat{u}_k(x_k) \in$$
$$\operatorname*{argmin}_{u_k \in U(x_k)} \mathbb{E}[g(x_k, x_{k+1}, u_k) + \tilde{J}_{k+1}(x_{k+1}, r_{k+1}) | x_{k+1} = \phi(x_k, u_k, \omega_k)]. \quad (6)$$

The policy set $U(x_k)$ is a finite set, so the best $\hat{u}_k$ is found by the direct comparison of a set of values. In general, the approximate function $\tilde{J}_k(\cdot, r_k)$ has a simple form and is easy to evaluate. Several practical architectures of $\tilde{J}_k(\cdot, r_k)$ are described below.

3.2 Approximation architectures

Designing and selecting suitable approximation architectures are important issues in NDP. For a given state, several representative features are extracted and serve as input to the approximation architecture. The output is usually a linear combination of features or a transformation via a neural network structure. We propose using the following three types of architecture:

1. *A neural network/multilayer perceptron architecture.* The input state x is encoded into a feature vector f with components $f_l(x), l = 1, 2, \ldots, L$, which represent the essential characteristics of the state. For example, in the fractionation radiotherapy problem, the average dose distribution and standard deviation of dose distribution are two important components of the feature vector associated with the state x, and it is a common practice to add the constant 1 as an additional feature. A concrete example of such a feature vector is given in Section 4.1.
   The feature vector is then linearly mapped with coefficients $r(j, l)$ to P 'hidden units' in a hidden layer,

$$\sum_{l=1}^{L} r(j, l) f_l(x), \; j = 1, 2, \ldots, P, \quad (7)$$

   as depicted in Figure 2.
   The values of each hidden unit are then input to a *sigmoidal function* that is differentiable and monotonically increasing. For example, the hyperbolic tangent function

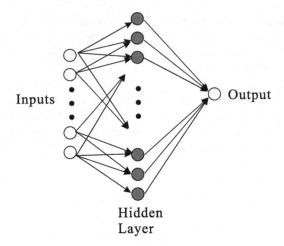

Fig. 2. An example of the structure of a neural network mapping.

$$\sigma(\xi) = \tanh(\xi) = \frac{e^\xi - e^{-\xi}}{e^\xi + e^{-\xi}},$$

or the logistic function

$$\sigma(\xi) = \frac{1}{1 + e^{-\xi}}$$

can be used. The sigmoidal functions should satisfy

$$-\infty < \lim_{\xi \to -\infty} \sigma(\xi) < \lim_{\xi \to \infty} \sigma(\xi) < \infty.$$

The output scalars of the sigmoidal function are linearly mapped again to generate one output value of the overall architecture,

$$\tilde{J}(x, r) = \sum_{j=1}^{P} r(j) \sigma \left(\sum_{l=1}^{L} r(j, l) f_l(x) \right). \tag{8}$$

Coefficients $r(j)$ and $r(j, l)$ in (7) are called the weights of the network. The weights are obtained from the training process of the algorithm.

2. *A feature extraction mapping.* An alternative architecture directly combines the feature vector $f(x)$ in a linear fashion, without using a neural network. The output of the architecture involves coefficients $r(l), l = 0, 1, 2, \ldots, L$,

$$\tilde{J}(x, r) = r(0) + \sum_{l=1}^{L} r(l) f_l(x). \tag{9}$$

An application of NDP that deals with playing strategies in a Tetris game involves such an architecture [2]. While this is attractive due to its simplicity, we did not find this architecture effective in our setting. The principal difficulty was that the iterative technique we used to determine r failed to converge.

3. *A heuristic mapping.* A third way to construct the approximate structure is based on existing heuristic controls. Heuristic controls are easy
to implement and produce decent solutions in a reasonable amount of
time. Although not optimal, some of the heuristic costs $H_u(x)$ are likely
to be fairly close to the optimal cost function $J(x)$. $H_u(x)$ is evaluated
by averaging results of simulations, in which policy u is applied in every
stage. In the heuristic mapping architecture, the heuristic costs are suitably weighted to obtain a good approximation of J. Given a state x and
heuristic controls $u_i, i = 1, 2, \ldots, I$, the approximate form of J is

$$\tilde{J}(x, r) = r(0) + \sum_{i=1}^{I} r(i) H_{u_i}(x), \tag{10}$$

where r is the overall tunable parameter vector of the architecture.
The more heuristic policies that are included in the training, the more
accurate the approximation is expected to be. With proper tuning of the
parameter vector r, we hope to obtain a policy that performs better than
all of the heuristic policies. However, each evaluation of $H_{u_i}(x)$ is potentially expensive.

3.3 Approximate policy iteration using Monte-Carlo simulation

The method we consider in this subsection is an approximate version of policy iteration. A sequence of policies $\{u_k\}$ is generated and the corresponding
approximate cost functions $\tilde{J}(x, r)$ are used in place of $J(x)$. The NDP algorithms are based on the architectures described previously. The training of
the parameter vector r for the architecture is performed using a combination
of Monte-Carlo simulation and least squares fitting.

The NDP algorithm we use is called *approximate policy iteration* (API)
using Monte-Carlo simulation. API alternates between approximate policy
evaluation steps (simulation) and policy improvement steps (training). Policies are iteratively updated from the outcomes of simulation. We expect the
policies will converge after several iterations, but there is no theoretical guarantee. Such an iteration process is illustrated in Figure 3.

Simulation step

Simulating sample trajectories starts with an initial state $x_0 = 0$, corresponding to no dose delivery. At the kth stage, an approximate cost-to-go function
$\tilde{J}_{k+1}(x_{k+1}, r_{k+1})$ for the next stage determines the policy $\hat{u}_k$ via the Equation
(6), using the knowledge of the transition probabilities. We can then simulate
x_{k+1} using the calculated $\hat{u}_k$ and a realization of ω_k. This process can be repeated to generate a collection of sample trajectories. In this simulation step,
the parameter vectors $r_k, k = 0, 1, \ldots, N - 1$, (which induce the policy $\hat{u}_k$)
remain fixed as all the sample trajectories are generated.

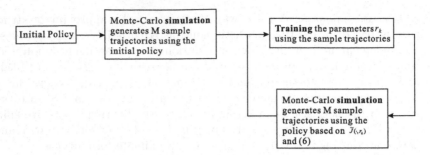

Fig. 3. Simulation and training in API. Starting with an initial policy, the Monte-Carlo simulation generates a number of sample trajectories. The sample costs at each stage are input into the training unit in which r_ks are updated by minimizing the least squares error. New sample trajectories are simulated using the policy based on the approximate structure $\tilde{J}(\cdot, r_k)$ and (6). This process is repeated.

Simulation generates sample trajectories $\{x_{0,i} = 0, x_{1,i}, \ldots, x_{N,i}\}, i = 1, 2, \ldots, M$. The corresponding sample cost-to-go for every transition state is equal to the cumulative instantaneous costs plus a final cost,

$$c(x_{k,i}) = \sum_{j=k}^{N-1} g(x_{j,i}, x_{j+1,i}, \hat{u}_j) + J_N(x_{N,i}).$$

Training step

In the training process, we evaluate the cost and update the r_k by solving a least squares problem at each stage $k = 0, 1, \ldots, N-1$,

$$\min_{r_k} \frac{1}{2} \sum_{i=1}^{M} |\tilde{J}_k(x_{k,i}, r_k) - c(x_{k,i})|^2. \tag{11}$$

The least squares problem (11) penalizes the difference of approximate cost-to-go estimation $\tilde{J}_k(x_{k,i}, r_k)$ and sample cost-to-go value $c(x_{k,i})$. It can be solved in various ways.

In practice, we divide the M generated trajectories into M_1 batches, with each batch containing M_2 trajectories.

$$M = M_1 * M_2.$$

The least squares formulation (11) is equivalently written as

$$\min_{r_k} \sum_{m=1}^{M_1} \left(\frac{1}{2} \sum_{x_{k,i} \in \text{Batch}_m} |\tilde{J}_k(x_{k,i}, r_k) - c(x_{k,i})|^2 \right). \tag{12}$$

We use a gradient-like method that processes each least squares term

$$\frac{1}{2} \sum_{x_{k,i} \in \text{Batch}_m} |\tilde{J}_k(x_{k,i}, r_k) - c(x_{k,i})|^2 \tag{13}$$

incrementally. The algorithm works as follows: Given a batch of sample state trajectories (M_2 trajectories), the parameter vector r_k is updated by

$$r_k := r_k - \gamma \sum_{x_{k,i} \in \text{Batch}_m} \nabla \tilde{J}_k(x_{k,i}, r_k) \left(\tilde{J}(x_{k,i}, r_k) - c(x_{k,i}) \right),$$
$$k = 0, 1, \ldots, N - 1. \tag{14}$$

Here γ is a stepsize length that should decrease monotonically as the number of batches used increases (see Proposition 3.8 in [3]). A suitable step length choice is $\gamma = \alpha/m, m = 1, 2, \ldots, M_1$, in the mth batch, where α is a constant scalar. The summation in the right-hand side of (14) is a gradient evaluation corresponding to (13) in the least squares formulation. The parametric vectors r_k are updated via the iteration (14), as a batch of trajectories become available. The incremental updating scheme is motivated by the stochastic gradient algorithm (more details are given in [3]).

In API, the r_ks are kept fixed until all the M sample trajectories are generated. In contrast to this, another form of the NDP algorithm, called *optimistic policy iteration* (OPI), updates the r_k more frequently, immediately after a batch of trajectories are generated. The intuition behind OPI is that the new changes on policies are incorporated rapidly. This 'optimistic' way of updating r_k is subject to further investigation.

Ferris and Voelker [10] applied a rollout policy to solve this same problem. The approximation is built by applying the particular control u at stage k and a control (base) policy at all future stages. This procedure ignores the training part of our algorithm. The rollout policy essentially suggests a simple form of

$$\tilde{J}(x) = H_{base}(x).$$

The simplification results in a biased estimation of $J(x)$, because the optimal cost-to-go function strictly satisfies $J(x) \leq H_{base}(x)$. In our new approach, we use an approximate functional architecture for the cost-to-go function, and the training process will determine the parameters in the architecture.

4 Computational experimentation

4.1 A simple example

We first experiment on a simple one dimensional fractionation problem with several variations of the approximating architectures described in the preceding section. As depicted in Fig. 4, the setting consists of a total of 15 voxels

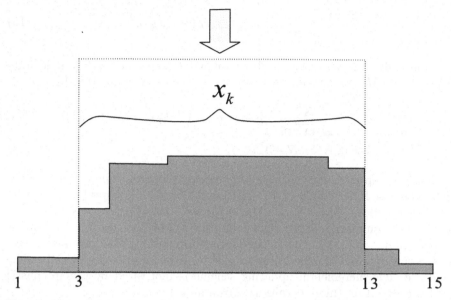

Fig. 4. A simple one-dimension problem. x_k is the dose distribution over voxels in the target: voxels $3, 4, \ldots, 13$.

$\{1, 2, \ldots, 15\}$, where the target voxel set, $\mathcal{T} = \{3, 4, \ldots, 13\}$, is located in the center. Dose is delivered to the target voxels, and due to the random positioning error of the patient, a portion of dose is delivered outside of the target. We assume a maximum shift of 2 voxels to the left or right.

In describing the cost function, our weighting scheme assigns relatively high weights on the target, and low weights elsewhere:

$$p(i) = \begin{cases} 10, \ i \in \mathcal{T}, \\ 1, \ \ i \notin \mathcal{T}. \end{cases}$$

Definitions of final error and one step error refer to (4) and (5).

For the target volume above, we also consider two different probability distributions for the random shift ω_k. In the low volatility examples, we have

$$\omega_k = \begin{cases} -2, \text{ with probability } 0.02 \\ -1, \text{ with probability } 0.08 \\ \ \ \ 0, \text{ with probability } 0.8 \\ \ \ \ 1, \text{ with probability } 0.08 \\ \ \ \ 2, \text{ with probability } 0.02, \end{cases}$$

for every stage k. The high volatility examples have

$$\omega_k = \begin{cases} -2, \text{ with probability } 0.05 \\ -1, \text{ with probability } 0.25 \\ 0, \text{ with probability } 0.4 \\ 1, \text{ with probability } 0.25 \\ 2, \text{ with probability } 0.05, \end{cases}$$

for every stage k. While it is hard to estimate the volatilities present in the given application, the results are fairly insensitive to these choices.

To apply the NDP approach, we should provide a rich collection of policies for the set $U(x_k)$. In our case, $U(x_k)$ consists of a total number of A modified reactive policies,

$$U(x_k) = \{u_{k,1}, u_{k,2}, \ldots, u_{k,A} | \, u_{k,i} = a_i \cdot \max(0, T - x_k)/(N - k)\}, \quad (15)$$

where a_i is a numerical scalar indicating an augmentation level to the standard reactive policy delivery; here $A = 5$ and

$$a = \{1, 1.4, 1.8, 2.2, 2.6\}.$$

We apply two of the approximation architectures in Section 3.2: the neural network/multilayer (NN) perceptron architecture and linear architecture using a heuristic mapping. The details follow.

1. API using Monte-Carlo simulation and neural network architecture.
   For the NN architecture, after experimentation with several different sets of features, we used the following six features $f_j(x), j = 1, 2, \ldots, 6$:
   a) Average dose distribution in the left rind of the target organ:

   $$\text{mean of } \{x(i), i = 3, 4, 5\}.$$

   b) Average dose distribution in the center of the target organ:

   $$\text{mean of } \{x(i), i = 6, 7, \ldots, 10\}.$$

   c) Average dose distribution in the right rind of the target organ:

   $$\text{mean of } \{x(i), i = 11, 12, 13\}.$$

   d) Standard deviation of the overall dose distribution in the target.
   e) Curvature of the dose distribution. The curvature is obtained by fitting a quadratic curve over the values $\{x_i, i = 3, 4, \ldots, 13\}$ and extracting the curvature.
   f) A constant feature $f_6(x) = 1$.
   In features (a)-(c), we distinguish the average dose on different parts of the structure, because the edges commonly have both underdose and overdose issues, while the center is delivered more accurately.

In the construction of neural network formulation, a hyperbolic tangent function was used as the sigmoidal mapping function. The neural network has 6 inputs (6 features), 8 hidden sigmoidal units, and 1 output, such that weight of neural network r_k is a vector of length 56.

In each simulation, a total of 10 policy iterations were performed. Running more policy iterations did not show further improvement. The initial policy used was the standard reactive policy u: $u_k = \max(0, T - x_k)/(N - k)$. Each iteration involved $M_1 = 15$ batches of sample trajectories, with $M_2 = 20$ trajectories in each batch to train the neural network.

To train the r_k in this approximate architecture, we started with $r_{k,0}$ as a vector of ones, and used an initial step length $\gamma = 0.5$.

2. API using Monte-Carlo simulation and the linear architecture of heuristic mapping.

Three heuristic policies were involved as base policies: (1) constant policy u_1: $u_{1,k} = T/N$, for all k; (2) standard reactive policy u_2: $u_{2,k} = \max(0, T - x_k)/(N - k)$, for all k; (3) modified reactive policy u_3 with the amplifying parameter $a = 2$ applied at all stages except the last one. For the stage $k = N - 1$, it simply delivers the residual dose:

$$u_{3,k} = \begin{cases} 2 \cdot \max(0, T - x_k)/(N - k), & k = 0, 1, \ldots, N - 2, \\ \max(0, T - x_k)/(N - k), & k = N - 1. \end{cases}$$

This third choice facilitates a more aggressive treatment in early stages. To evaluate the heuristic cost $H_{u_i}(x_k), i = 1, 2, 3$, 100 sub-trajectories starting with x_k were generated for periods k to N. The training scheme was analogous to the above method. A total of 10 policy iterations were performed. The policy used in the first iteration was the standard reactive policy. All iterations involved $M_1 = 15$ batches of sample trajectories, with $M_2 = 20$ trajectories in each batch, resulting in a total of 300 trajectories. Running the heuristic mapping architecture entails a great deal of computation, because it requires evaluating the heuristic costs by sub-simulations.

The fractionation radiotherapy problem is solved using both techniques with $N = 3, 4, 5, 10, 14$ and 20 stages. Figure 5 shows performance of API using a heuristic mapping architecture in a low volatility case. The starting policy is the standard reactive policy, that has an expected error (cost) of 0.48 (over $M = 300$ sample trajectories). The policies u_k converge after around 7 policy iterations, taking around 20 minutes on a PIII 1.4GHz machine. After the training, the expected error decreases to 0.30, which is reduced by about 40% compared to the standard reactive policy.

The main results of training and simulation with two probability distributions are plotted in Figure 6. This one-dimension example is small, but the revealed patterns are informative. For each plot, the results of the constant policy, reactive policy and NDP policy are displayed. Due to the significant randomness in the high volatility case, it is more likely to induce underdose in the rind of target, which is penalized heavily with our weighting scheme. Thus,

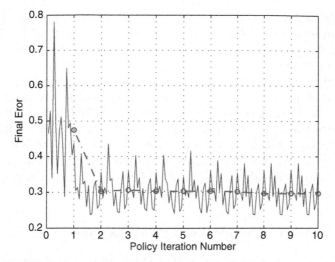

Fig. 5. Performance of API using heuristic cost mapping architecture, $N = 20$. For every iteration, we plot the average (over $M_2 = 20$ trajectories) of each of $M_1 = 15$ batches. The broken line represents the mean cost in each iteration.

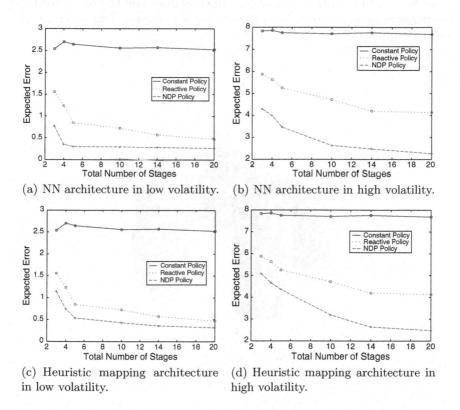

(a) NN architecture in low volatility.   (b) NN architecture in high volatility.

(c) Heuristic mapping architecture in low volatility.   (d) Heuristic mapping architecture in high volatility.

Fig. 6. Comparing the constant, reactive and NDP policies in low and high volatility cases.

as volatility increases, so does the error. Note that in this one-dimensional problem, an ideal total amount of dose delivered to target is 11, which can be compared with the values on the vertical axes of the plots (which are multiplied by the vector p).

Comparing the figures, we note remarkable similarities. Common to all examples is the poor performance of the constant policy. The reactive policy performs better than the constant policy, but not as well as the NDP policy in either architecture. The constant policy does not change much with number of total fractions. The level of improvement depends on the NDP approximate structure used. The NN architecture performs better than the heuristic mapping architecture when N is small. When N is large, they do not show significant difference.

4.2 A real patient example: head and neck tumor

In this subsection, we apply our NDP techniques to a real patient problem — a head and neck tumor. In the head and neck tumor scenario, the tumor volume covers a total of 984 voxels in space. As noted in Figure 7, the tumor is circumscribed by two critical organs: the mandible and the spinal cord. We will perform analogous techniques as in the above simple example. The weight setting is the same:

$$p(i) = \begin{cases} 10, i \in \mathcal{T}, \\ 1, \ i \notin \mathcal{T}. \end{cases}$$

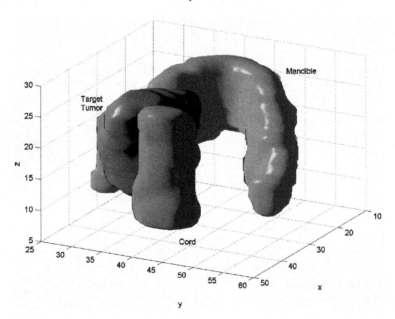

Fig. 7. Target tumor, cord and mandible in the head and neck problem scenario.

In our problem setting, we do not distinguish between critical organs and other normal tissue. In reality, a physician also takes into account radiation damage to the surrounding critical organs. For this reason, a higher penalty weight is usually assigned on these organs.

ω_k are now three-dimension random vectors. By assumption of independence of each component direction, we have

$$Pr(\omega_k = [i, j, k]) = Pr(\omega_{k,x} = i) \cdot Pr(\omega_{k,y} = j) \cdot Pr(\omega_{k,z} = k). \qquad (16)$$

In the low and high volatility cases, each component of ω_k follows a discrete distribution (also with a maximum shift of two voxels),

$$\omega_{k,i} = \begin{cases} -2, \text{ with probability } 0.01 \\ -1, \text{ with probability } 0.06 \\ 0, \text{ with probability } 0.86 \\ 1, \text{ with probability } 0.06 \\ 2, \text{ with probability } 0.01, \end{cases}$$

and

$$\omega_{k,i} = \begin{cases} -2, \text{ with probability } 0.05 \\ -1, \text{ with probability } 0.1 \\ 0, \text{ with probability } 0.7 \\ 1, \text{ with probability } 0.1 \\ 2, \text{ with probability } 0.05. \end{cases}$$

We adjust the $\omega_{k,i}$ by smaller amounts than in the one dimension problem, because the overall probability is the product of each component (16); the resulting volatility therefore grows.

For each stage, $U(x_k)$ is a set of modified reactive policies, whose augmentation levels include

$$a = \{1, 1.5, 2, 2.5, 3\}.$$

For the stage $k = N - 1$ (when there are two stages to go), setting the augmentation level $a > 2$ is equivalent to delivering more than the residual dose, which is unnecessary for treatment. In fact, the NDP algorithm will ignore these choices.

The approximate policy iteration algorithm uses the same two architectures as in Section 4.1. However, for the neural network architecture, we need an extended 12 dimensional input feature space:

(a) Features 1-7 are the mean values of the dose distribution of the left, right, up, down, front, back and center parts of the tumor.
(b) Feature 8 is the standard deviation of dose distribution in the tumor volume.

(c) Features 9-11. We extract the dose distribution on three lines through the center of the tumor. Lines are from left to right, from up to down, and from front to back. Features 9-11 are the estimated curvature of the dose distribution on the three lines.

(d) Feature 12 is a constant feature, set as 1.

In the neural network architecture, we build 1 hidden layer, with 16 hidden sigmoidal units. Therefore, each r_k for $\tilde{J}(x, r_k)$ is of length 208.

We still use 10 policy iterations. (Later experimentation shows that 5 policy iterations are enough for policy convergence.) In each iteration, simulation generates a total of 300 sample trajectories that are grouped in $M_1 = 15$ batches of sample trajectories, with $M_2 = 20$ in each batch, to train the parameter r_k.

One thing worth mentioning here is the initial step length scaler γ in (14) is set to a much smaller value in the 3D problem. In the head and neck case, we set $\gamma = 0.00005$ as compared to $\gamma = 0.5$ in the one dimension example. A plot, Figure 8, shows the reduction of expected error as the number of policy iteration increases.

The alternative architecture for $\tilde{J}(x, r)$ using a linear combination of heuristic costs is implemented precisely as in the one dimension example.

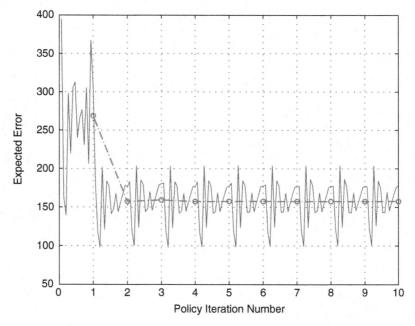

Fig. 8. Performance of API using neural-network architecture, $N = 11$. For every iteration, we plot the average (over $M_2 = 20$ trajectories) of each of $M_1 = 15$ batches. The broken line represents the mean cost in each policy iteration.

The overall performance of this second architecture is very slow, due to the large amount of work in evaluation of the heuristic costs. It spends a considerable time in the simulation process generating sample sub-trajectories. To save computation time, we propose an approximate way of evaluating each candidate policy in (6). The expected cost associated with policy u_k is

$$\mathbb{E}[g(x_k, x_{k+1}, u_k) + \tilde{J}_{k+1}(x_{k+1}, r_{k+1})]$$
$$= \sum_{\omega_{k,1}=-2}^{2} \sum_{\omega_{k,2}=-2}^{2} \sum_{\omega_{k,2}=-2}^{2} Pr(\omega_k)[g(x_k, x_{k+1}, u_k) + \tilde{J}_{k+1}(x_{k+1}, r_{k+1})].$$

For a large portion of ω_k, the value of $Pr(\omega_k)$ almost vanishes to zero when it makes a two-voxel shift in each direction. Thus, we only compute the sum of costs over a subset of possible ω_k,

$$\sum_{\omega_{k,1}=-1}^{1} \sum_{\omega_{k,2}=-1}^{1} \sum_{\omega_{k,2}=-1}^{1} Pr(\omega_k)[g(x_k, x_{k+1}, u_k) + \tilde{J}_{k+1}(x_{k+1}, r_{k+1})].$$

A straightforward calculation shows that we reduce a total of $125(= 5^3)$ evaluations of state x_{k+1} to $27(= 3^3)$. The final time involved in training the architecture is around 10 hours.

Again, we plot the results of constant policy, reactive policy and NDP policy in the same figure. We still investigate on the cases where $N = 3, 4, 5, 14, 20$. As we can observe in all sub-figures in Figure 9, the constant policy still performs the worst in both high and low volatility cases. The reactive policy is better and the NDP policy is best. As the total number of stages increases, the constant policy remains almost at the same level, but the reactive and NDP continue to improve. The poor constant policy is a consequence of significant underdose near the edge of the target.

The two approximating architectures perform more or less the same, though the heuristic mapping architecture takes significantly more time to train. Focusing on the low volatility cases, Figure 9 (a) and (c), we see the heuristic mapping architecture outperforms the NN architecture when N is small, i.e., $N = 3, 4, 5, 10$. When $N = 20$, the expected error is reduced to the lowest, about 50% from reactive policy to NDP policy. When N is small, the improvement ranges from 30% to 50%. When the volatility is high, it undoubtedly induces more error than in low volatility. Not only the expected error, but the variance escalates to a large value as well.

For the early fractions of the treatment, the NDP algorithm intends to select aggressive policies, i.e., the augmentation level $a > 2$, while in the later stage time, it intends to choose more conservative polices. Since the weighting factor for target voxels is 10, aggressive policies are preferred in the early stage because they leave room to correct the delivery error on the target in the later stages. However, it may be more likely to cause delivery error on the normal tissue.

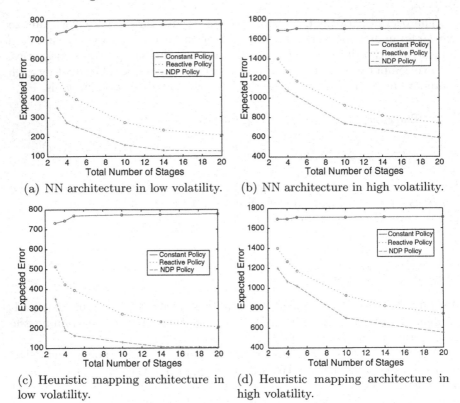

(a) NN architecture in low volatility.   (b) NN architecture in high volatility.

(c) Heuristic mapping architecture in low volatility.   (d) Heuristic mapping architecture in high volatility.

Fig. 9. Head and neck problem — comparing constant, reactive and NDP policies in two probability distributions.

4.3 Discussion

The number of candidate policies used in training is small. Once we have the optimal r_k after simulation and training procedures, we can select u_k from an extended set of policies $U(x_k)$ (via (6)) using the approximate cost-to-go functions $\tilde{J}(x, r_k)$, improving upon the current results.

For instance, we can introduce a new class of policies that cover a wider delivery region. This class of clinically favored policies includes a safety margin around the target. The policies deliver the same dose to voxels in the margin as delivered to the nearest voxels in the target. As an example policy in the class, a constant-w1 policy (where 'w1' means '1 voxel wider') is an extension of the constant policy, covering a 1-voxel thick margin around the target. As in the one-dimensional example in Section 4.1, the constant-w1 policy is defined as:

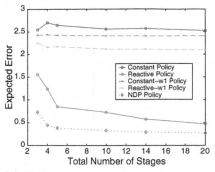 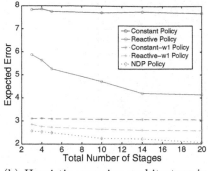

(a) Heuristic mapping architecture in low volatility.

(b) Heuristic mapping architecture in high volatility.

Fig. 10. In the one-dimensional problem, NDP policies with extended policy set $U(x_k)$.

$$u_k(i) = \begin{cases} T(i)/N, & \text{for } i \in \mathcal{T}, \\ T(3)/N = T(13)/N, & \text{for } i = 2 \text{ or } 14, \\ 0, & \text{elsewhere,} \end{cases}$$

where the voxel set $\{2, 14\}$ represents the margin of the target. The reactive-w1 policies and the modified reactive-w1 policies are defined accordingly. (We prefer to use 'w1' policies rather than 'w2' policies because 'w1' policies are observed to be uniformly better.)

The class of 'w1' policies are preferable to apply in the high volatility case, but not in the low volatility case (see Figure 10). For the high volatility case, the policies reduce the underdose error significantly, which is penalized 10 times as heavy as the overdose error, easily compensating for the overdose error they introduce outside of the target. In the low volatility case, when the underdose is not as severe, they inevitably introduce redundant overdose error.

The NDP technique was applied to an enriched policy set $U(x_k)$, including the constant, constant-w1, reactive, reactive-w1, modified reactive and modified reactive-w1 policies. It automatically selected an appropriate policy at each stage based on the approximated cost-to-go function, and outperformed every component policy in the policy set. In Figure 10, we show the result of the one-dimensional example using the heuristic mapping architecture for NDP. As we have observed, in the low volatility case, the NDP policy tends to be the reactive or the modified reactive policy, while in the high volatility case is more likely to be the reactive-w1 or the modified reactive-w1 policy. Comparing to the NDP policies in Figure 6, we see that increasing the choices of policies in $U(x_k)$, the NDP policy generates a lower expected error.

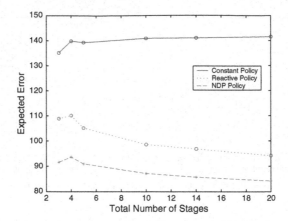

Fig. 11. Head and neck problem. Using API with a neural network architecture, in a low volatility case, with identical weight on the target and normal tissue.

Another question concerns the amount of difference that occurs when switching to another weighting scheme. Setting a high weighting factor on the target is rather arbitrary. This will also influence the NDP in selecting policies. In addition, we changed the setting of weighting scheme to

$$p(i) = \begin{cases} 1, \, i \in \mathcal{T}, \\ 1, \, i \notin \mathcal{T}, \end{cases}$$

and ran the experiment on the real example (Section 4.2) again. In Figure 11, we discovered the same pattern of results, while this time, all the error curves were scaled down accordingly. The difference between constant and reactive policy decreased. The NDP policy showed an improvement of around 12% over the reactive policy when $N = 10$.

We even tested the weighting scheme

$$p(i) = \begin{cases} 1, \;\; i \in \mathcal{T}, \\ 10, \, i \notin \mathcal{T}, \end{cases}$$

which reverted the importance of the target and the surrounding tissue. It resulted in a very small amount of delivered dose in the earlier stages, and at the end the target was severely underdosed. The result was reasonable because the NDP policy was cautious to deliver any dose outside of the target at each stage.

5 Conclusion

Solving an optimal on-line planning strategy in fractionated radiation treatment is quite complex. In this paper, we set up a dynamic model for the day-to-day planning problem. We assume that the probability distribution of patient motion can be estimated by means of prior inspection. In fact, our experimentation on both high and low volatility cases displays very similar patterns.

Although methods such as dynamic programming obtain exact solutions, the computation is intractable. We exploit neuro-dynamic programming tools to derive approximate DP solutions that can be solved with much fewer computational resources. The API algorithm we apply iteratively switches between Monte-Carlo simulation steps and training steps, whereby the feature based approximating architectures of the cost-to-go function are enhanced as the algorithm proceeds. The computational results are based on a finite policy set for training. In fact, the final approximate cost-to-go structures can be used to facilitate selection from a larger set of candidate policies extended from the training set.

We jointly compare the on-line policies with an off-line constant policy that simply delivers a fixed dose amount in each fraction of treatment. The on-line policies are shown to be significantly better than the constant policy in terms of total expected delivery error. In most of the cases, the expected error is reduced by more than half. The NDP policy performs preferentially, enhancing the reactive policy for all our tests. Future work needs to address further timing improvement.

We have tested two approximation architectures. One uses a neural network and the other is based on existing heuristic policies, both of which perform similarly. The heuristic mapping architecture is slightly better than the neural network based architecture, but it takes significantly more computational time to evaluate. As these examples have demonstrated, neuro-dynamic programming is a promising supplement to heuristics in discrete dynamic optimization.

References

1. D. P. Bertsekas. *Dynamic Programming and Optimal Control.* Athena Scientific, Belmont, Massachusetts, 1995.
2. D. P. Bertsekas and S. Ioffe. Temporal differences-based policy iteration and applications in neuro-dynamic programming. Technical report, Lab. for Information and Decision Systems, MIT, 1996.
3. D. P. Bertsekas and J. N. Tsitsiklis. *Neuro-Dynamic Programming.* Athena Scientific, Belmont, Massachusetts, 1996.
4. J. R. Birge and R. Louveaux. *Introduction to Stochastic Programming.* Springer, New York, 1997.
5. M. Birkner, D. Yan, M. Alber, J. Liang, and F. Nusslin. Adapting inverse planning to patient and organ geometrical variation: Algorithm and implementation. *Medical Physics*, 30:2822–2831, 2003.
6. Th. Bortfeld. Current status of IMRT: physical and technological aspects. *Radiotherapy and Oncology*, 61:291–304, 2001.

7. C. L. Creutzberg, G. V. Althof, M. de Hooh, A. G. Visser, H. Huizenga, A. Wijnmaalen, and P. C. Levendag. A quality control study of the accuracy of patient positioning in irradiation of pelvic fields. *International Journal of Radiation Oncology, Biology and Physics*, 34:697–708, 1996.

8. M. C. Ferris, J.-H. Lim, and D. M. Shepard. Optimization approaches for treatment planning on a Gamma Knife. *SIAM Journal on Optimization*, 13:921–937, 2003.

9. M. C. Ferris, J.-H. Lim, and D. M. Shepard. Radiosurgery treatment planning via nonlinear programming. *Annals of Operations Research*, 119:247–260, 2003.

10. M. C. Ferris and M. M. Voelker. Fractionation in radiation treatment planning. *Mathematical Programming B*, 102:387–413, 2004.

11. A. Gosavi. *Simulation-Based Optimization: Parametric Optimization Techniques and Reinforcement Learning*. Kluwer Academic Publishers, Norwell, MA, USA, 2003.

12. M. A. Hunt, T. E. Schultheiss, G. E. Desobry, M. Hakki, and G. E. Hanks. An evaluation of setup uncertainties for patients treated to pelvic fields. *International Journal of Radiation Oncology, Biology and Physics*, 32:227–233, 1995.

13. P. Kall and S. W. Wallace. *Stochastic Programming*. John Wiley & Sons, Chichester, 1994.

14. K. M. Langen and T. L. Jones. Organ motion and its management. *International Journal of Radiation Oncology, Biology and Physics*, 50:265–278, 2001.

15. J. G. Li and L. Xing. Inverse planning incorporating organ motion. *Medical Physics*, 27:1573–1578, 2000.

16. A. Niemierko. Optimization of 3D radiation therapy with both physical and biological end points and constraints. *International Journal of Radiation Oncology, Biology and Physics*, 23:99–108, 1992.

17. W. Schlegel and A. Mahr, editors. *3D Conformal Radiation Therapy - A Multimedia Introduction to Methods and Techniques*. Springer-Verlag, Berlin, 2001.

18. D. M. Shepard, M. C. Ferris, G. Olivera, and T. R. Mackie. Optimizing the delivery of radiation to cancer patients. *SIAM Review*, 41:721–744, 1999.

19. J. Unkelback and U. Oelfke. Inclusion of organ movements in IMRT treatment planning via inverse planning based on probability distributions. *Institute of Physics Publishing, Physics in Medicine and Biology*, 49:4005–4029, 2004.

20. J. Unkelback and U. Oelfke. Incorporating organ movements in inverse planning: Assessing dose uncertainties by Bayesian inference. *Institute of Physics Publishing, Physics in Medicine and Biology*, 50:121–139, 2005.

21. L. J. Verhey. Immobilizing and positioning patients for radiotherapy. *Seminars in Radiation Oncology*, 5:100–113, 1995.

22. M. M. Voelker. *Optimization of Slice Models*. PhD thesis, University of Wisconsin, Madison, Wisconsin, December 2002.

23. S. Webb. *The Physics of Conformal Radiotherapy: Advances in Technology*. Institute of Physics Publishing Ltd., 1997.

Randomized algorithms for mixed matching and covering in hypergraphs in 3D seed reconstruction in brachytherapy

Helena Fohlin[2], Lasse Kliemann[1]*, and Anand Srivastav[1]

[1] Institut für Informatik
   Christian–Albrechts–Universität zu Kiel
   Christian-Albrechts-Platz 4, D–24098 Kiel, Germany
   {lki,asr}@numerik.uni-kiel.de
[2] Department of Oncology
   Linköping University Hospital
   581 85 Linköping, Sweden
   helena.fohlin@lio.se

Summary. Brachytherapy is a radiotherapy method for cancer. In its low dose radiation (LDR) variant a number of radioactive implants, so-called seeds, are inserted into the affected organ through an operation. After the implantation, it is essential to determine the locations of the seeds in the organ. A common method is to take three X-ray photographs from different angles; the seeds show up on the X-ray photos as small white lines. In order to reconstruct the three-dimensional configuration from these X-ray photos, one has to determine which of these white lines belong to the same seed. We model the problem as a mixed packing and covering hypergraph optimization problem and present a randomized approximation algorithm based on linear programming. We analyse the worst-case performance of the algorithm by discrete probabilistic methods and present results for data of patients with prostate cancer from the university clinic of Schleswig-Holstein, Campus Kiel. These examples show an almost optimal performance of the algorithm which presently cannot be matched by the theoretical analysis.

Keywords: Prostate cancer, brachytherapy, seed reconstruction, combinatorial optimization, randomized algorithms, probabilistic methods, concentration inequalities.

1 Introduction

Brachytherapy is a method developed in the 1980s for cancer radiation in organs like the prostate, lung, or breast. At the Clinic of Radiotherapy (radiooncology), University Clinic of Schleswig-Holstein, Campus Kiel, among others,

---

* Supported by the Deutsche Forschungsgemeinschaft (DFG), Grant Sr7-3.

low dose radiation therapy (LDR therapy) for the treatment of prostate cancer is applied, where 25-80 small radioactive seeds are implanted in the affected organ. They have to be placed so that the tumor is exposed with sufficiently high radiation and adjacent healthy tissue is exposed to as low a radiation dose as possible. Unavoidably, the seeds can move due to blood circulation, movements of the organ, etc. For the quality control of the treatment plan, the locations of the seeds after the operation have to be checked. This is done by taking usually 3 X-ray photographs from three different angles (so-called 3-film technique). On the films the seeds appear as white lines. To determine the positions of the seeds in the organ the task now is to match the three different images (lines) representing the same seed.

1.1 Previous and related work

The 3-film technique was independently applied by Rosenthal and Nath [22], Biggs and Kelley [9] and Altschuler, Findlay, Epperson [2], while Siddon and Chin [12] applied a special 2-film technique that took the seed endpoints as image points rather than the seed centers. The algorithms invoked in these papers are matching heuristics justified by experimental results. New algorithmic efforts were taken in the last 5 years. Tubic, Zaccarin, Beaulieu and Pouliot [8] used simulated annealing, Todor, Cohen, Amols and Zaider [3] combined several heuristic approaches, and Lam, Cho, Marks and Narayanan [13] introduced the so-called Hough transform, a standard method in image processing and computer vision for the seed reconstruction problem. Recently, Narayanan, Cho and Marks [14] also addressed the problem of reconstruction with an incomplete data set. These papers essentially focus on the improvement of the geometric projections. From the mathematical programming side, branch-and-bound was applied by Balas and Saltzman [7] and Brogan [10]. These papers provide the link to integer programming models of the problem.

None of these papers give a mathematical analysis or provable performance guarantee of the algorithms in use. In particular, since different projection techniques essentially result in different objective functions, it would be desirable to have an algorithm which is independent of the specific projection technique and thus is applicable to all such situations. Furthermore, it is today considered a challenging task in algorithmic discrete mathematics and theoretical computer science to give fast algorithms for NP-hard problems, which provably (or at least in practice) approximate the optimal solution. This is sometimes a fast alternative to branch-and-bound methods.

A comprehensive treatment of randomized rounding algorithms for packing and covering integer programs has been given by Srivastav [27] and Srivastav and Stangier [28].

The presented algorithm has also been studied in [15]. Experimental results on an algorithm based on a different LP formulation combined with a visualization technique have recently been published [26].

1.2 Our contribution

In this paper we model the seed reconstruction problem as a minimum-weight perfect matching problem in a hypergraph: we consider a complete 3-uniform hypergraph, where its nodes are the seed images on the three films, and each of its hyperedges contains three nodes (one from each X-ray photo). We define a weight function for the hyperedges, which is close to zero if the three lines from a hyperedge belong to the same seed and increases otherwise. The goal is to find a matching, i.e., a subset of pairwise disjoint hyperedges, so that all nodes are covered and the total weight of these hyperedges is minimum. This is nothing other than the minimum-weight perfect matching problem in a hypergraph. Since this problem generalizes the NP-hard 3-dimensional assignment problem (see [16]), it is NP-hard as well. Thus we can only hope to find an algorithm which solves the problem approximately in polynomial time, unless $P = NP$.

We model the problem as an integer linear program. To solve this integer program, an algorithm based on the so-called randomized rounding scheme introduced by Raghavan and Thompson [24] is designed and applied. This algorithm is not only very fast, but accessible at least in part for a mathematical rigorous analysis. We give a partial analysis of the algorithm combining probabilistic and combinatorial methods, which shows that in the worst-case the solution produced is in some strong sense close to a minimum-weight perfect matching. The heart of the analytical methods are tools from probability theory, like large deviation inequalities. All in all, our algorithm points towards a mathematically rigorous analysis of heuristics for the seed reconstruction problem and is practical as well. Furthermore, the techniques developed here are promising for an analysis of mixed integer packing and covering problems, which are of independent interest in discrete optimization.

Moreover, we show that an implementation of our algorithm is very effective on a set of patient data from the Clinic of Radiotherapy, University Clinic of Schleswig-Holstein, Campus Kiel. In fact, the algorithm for a certain choice of parameters outputs optimal or nearly optimal solutions where only a few seeds are unmatched. It is interesting that the practical results are much better than the results of the theoretical analysis indicate. Here we have the challenging situation of closing the gap between the theoretical analysis and the good practical performance, which should be addressed in future work.

In conclusion, while in previous work on the seed reconstruction problem only heuristics were used, this paper is a first step in designing mathematical analyzable *and* practically efficient algorithms.

The paper is organized as follows.

In Section 2 we describe the seed reconstruction problem more precisely and give a mathematical model. For this we introduce the notion of (b, k)-matching which generalizes the notions of b-matching in hypergraphs and partial k-covering in hypergraphs. In fact, a (b, k)-matching is a b-matching, i.e., a subset of hyperedges such that no node is incident in more than b of them, covering at least k nodes. So for a hypergraph with n nodes, $(1, n)$-matching is a perfect matching problem. Furthermore, some large deviation inequalities are listed as well.

In Section 3 we give an integer linear programming formulation for the (b, k)-matching problem and state the randomized rounding algorithm. This algorithm solves the linear programming (LP) relaxation up to optimality and then generates an integer solution by picking edges with the probabilities given by the optimal LP-solution. After this procedure we remove edges in a greedy way to get a feasible b-matching.

In Section 4 we analyze the algorithm with probabilistic tools.

In Section 5 we test the practical performance of the algorithm on real patient data for five patients treated in the Clinic of Radiotherapy in Kiel. The algorithm is implemented in C^{++}, and is iterated for each patient data set 100 times. For most of the patients all seeds are matched if we choose good values of the parameters, i.e., letting them be close to the values enforcing a minimum-weight perfect matching. The algorithm is very fast: within a few seconds of CPU time on a PC, it delivers the solution.

2 Hypergraph matching model of 3D seed reconstruction

Brachytherapy is a cancer radiation therapy developed in the 1980s. In the low dose variant of brachytherapy, about 25 to 80 small radioactive implants called seeds are placed in organs like the prostate, lung or breast, and remain there. A seed is a titan cylinder of length approximately 4.5 mm encapsulating radioactive material like Iod-125 or Pd-103.

The method allows an effective continuous radiation of tumor tissue with a relatively low dose for a long time in which radiation is delivered at a very short distance to the tumor by placing the radioactive source in the affected organ. Today it is a widely spread technique and an alternative to the usual external radiation. A benefit for the patient is certainly that he/she does not have to suffer from a long treatment with various radiation sessions. For the treatment of prostate cancer, brachytherapy has been reported as a very effective method [6]. At the Clinic of Radiotherapy, University Clinic of Schleswig-Holstein, Campus Kiel, brachytherapy has become the standard radiation treatment of prostate cancer.

2.1 The optimization problem

In LDR brachytherapy with seeds two mathematical optimization problems play a central role:

Placement problem

The most important problem is to determine a minimum number of seeds along with their placement in the organ. The placement must be such that

a) the tumor tissue is exposed with sufficient dose avoiding cold spots (regions with insufficient radiation) and hot spots (regions with too much radiation) and

b) normal tissue or critical regions like the urethra are exposed with a minimum possible, medical tolerable dose.

The problem thus appears as a combination of several NP-hard multicriteria optimization problems, e.g., set covering and facility location with restricted areas. Since the dose distribution emitted by the seeds is highly nonlinear, the problem is further complicated beyond set covering with regular geometric objects, like balls, ellipsoids, etc. An intense research has been done in this area in the last 10 years. Among the most effective placement tools are the mixed-integer programming methods proposed by Lee [20]. At the Clinic of Radiotherapy, University Clinic of Schleswig-Holstein, Campus Kiel, a commercial placement software (VariSeed® of the company VARIAN) is applied. The software offers a two-film and a three-film technique. According to the manual of the software, the three-film technique is an ad hoc extension of the two-film technique of Chin and Siddon [12].

3D seed reconstruction problem

After the operative implantation of the seeds, due to blood circulation and movements of the organ or patient, the seeds can change their original position. Usually 1-2 hours after the operation a determination of the actual seed positions in the organ is necessary in order to control the quality and to take further steps. In the worst case a short high dose radiation (HDR brachytherapy) has to be conducted.

The seed locations are determined by three X-ray films of the organ taken from three different angles, see Figures 1, 2, and 3. This technique was introduced by Amols and Rosen [4] in 1981. The advantage of the 3-film technique compared with the 2-film technique is that it seems to be less ambiguous in identifying seed locations. So, each film shows the seeds from a different 3-dimensional perspective. The task is to determine the location of the seeds in the organ by matching seed images on the three films.

To formalize the seed reconstruction problem, an appropriate geometrical measure as a cost function for matching three seed images from each film is introduced. We now show how the cost function is computed for the upper endpoint of the seed (see Figure 4). The cost of the lower endpoint is calculated in the same way.

For the three seed images we have three lines P_1, P_2, P_3 connecting the lower respectively upper endpoint of the seed images with the X-ray source. We determine the shortest connections between the lines P_i and P_j for all i, j. Let $r_i = (x_i, y_i, z_i)$ be the centers of the shortest connections and let $\overline{x}, \overline{y}, \overline{z}$ be the mean values of the x, y, z coordinate of r_1, r_2, r_3. We define the standard deviation

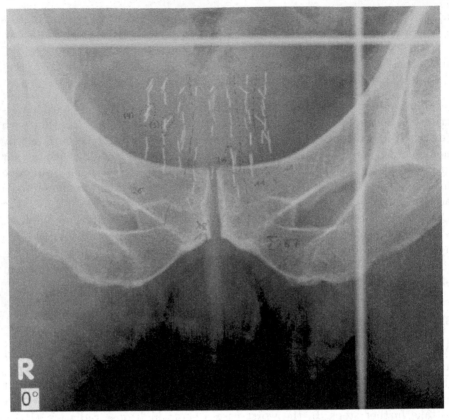

Fig. 1. X-ray, 0 degrees. Figures 1, 2, and 3 were provided by Dr. F.-A. Siebert, Clinic of Radiotherapy, University Clinic of Schleswig-Holstein, Campus Kiel, Kiel, Germany.

$$\Delta r = \sqrt{\frac{1}{3}\sum_{i=1}^{3}(x_i - \overline{x})^2} + \sqrt{\frac{1}{3}\sum_{i=1}^{3}(y_i - \overline{y})^2} + \sqrt{\frac{1}{3}\sum_{i=1}^{3}(z_i - \overline{z})^2}.$$

The cost for the upper (respectively lower) endpoint of *any* choice of three seed images from the three X-ray photos is the Δr of the associated lines. It is clear that Δr is close to zero if the three seed images represent the same seed.

The *total cost* for three seed images is the sum of the standard deviation Δr for the upper endpoint and the standard deviation for the lower endpoint.[3]

An alternative cost measure can be the area spanned by the triangle r_1, r_2, r_3. But in this paper this cost function is not considered.

---

[3] By appropriate scaling Δr to $\Delta r / \alpha$, with some $\alpha \geq 1$, one can assume that the total cost is in $[0, 1]$.

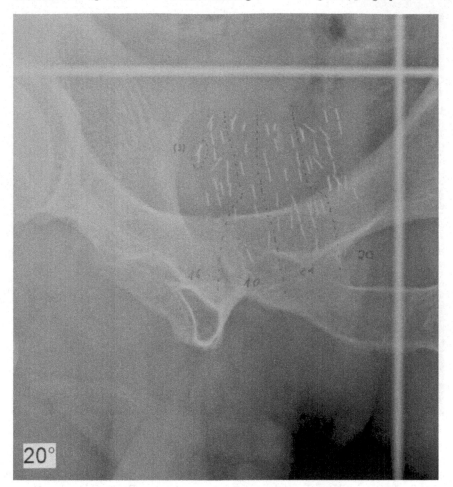

Fig. 2. X-ray, 20 degrees.

If the cost function is well posed, the optimal solution of the problem should be in one-to-one correspondence to the real seed locations in the organ. Thus the problem reduces to a three-dimensional assignment (or matching) problem, where we minimize the cost of the matching. In the literature the problem is also noted as the AP3 problem, which is NP-hard. Thus under the hypothesis $P \neq NP$, we cannot expect an efficient, i.e., polynomial time algorithm solving the problem to optimality.

2.2 Hypergraph matching and seed reconstruction

We use the standard notion of graphs and hypergraphs. A finite graph $G = (V, E)$ is a pair of a finite set V (the set of vertices or nodes) and a subset $E \subseteq \binom{V}{2}$, where $\binom{V}{2}$ denotes the set of all $2-$element subsets of V. The

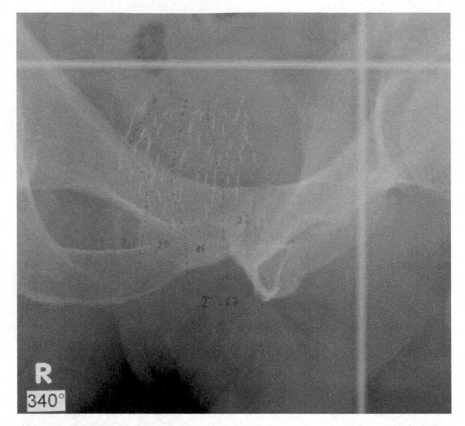

Fig. 3. X-ray, 340 degrees.

elements of E are called edges. A hypergraph (or set system) $\mathcal{H} = (V, \mathcal{E})$ is a pair of a finite set V and a subset $\mathcal{E}$ of the power set $\mathcal{P}(V)$. The elements of $\mathcal{E}$ are called hyperedges.

Let $\mathcal{H} = (V, \mathcal{E})$ be a hypergraph. For $v \in V$ we define

$$deg(v) := |\{E \in \mathcal{E}; v \in E\}| \quad \text{and} \quad \Delta = \Delta(\mathcal{H}) := \max_{v \in V} deg(v).$$

We call $deg(v)$ the vertex-degree of v and $\Delta(\mathcal{H})$ is the maximum vertex degree of $\mathcal{H}$.

The hypergraph $\mathcal{H}$ is called $r-$regular respectively $s-$uniform, if $\deg(v) = r$ for all $v \in V$ respectively $|E| = s$ for all $E \in \mathcal{E}$. It is convenient to order the vertices and hyperedges, $V = \{v_1, \cdots, v_n\}$ and $\mathcal{E} = \{E_1, \cdots, E_m\}$, and to identify vertices and edges with their indices. The hyperedge-vertex incidence matrix of a hypergraph $\mathcal{H} = (V, \mathcal{E})$, with $V = \{v_1, \cdots, v_n\}$ and $\mathcal{E} = \{E_1, \cdots, E_m\}$, is the matrix $A = (a_{ij}) \in \{0, 1\}^{m \times n}$, where $a_{ij} = 1$ if $v_j \in E_i$, and 0 else. Sometimes the vertex-hyperedge incidence matrix A^T is used.

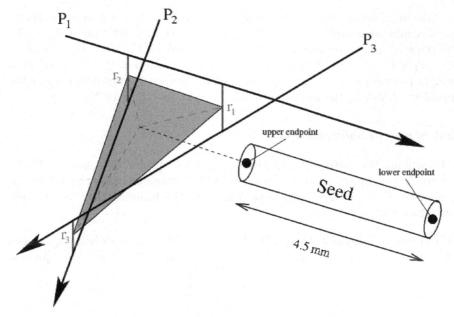

Fig. 4. Cost function for the upper endpoint.

We proceed to the formulation of a mathematical model for the seed re-construction problem.

Definition 1. *Let $\mathcal{H} = (V, \mathcal{E})$ be a hypergraph with $|V| = n, |\mathcal{E}| = m$.*
Let $w : \mathcal{E} \to \mathbb{Q} \cap [0, 1]$ be a weight function. Let $b, k \in \mathbb{N}$.

(i) A b-matching in $\mathcal{H}$ is a subset $\mathcal{E}^* \subseteq \mathcal{E}$ such that each $v \in V$ is contained in at most b edges of $\mathcal{E}^*$.
(ii) A (b, k)-matching $\mathcal{E}^*$ is a b-matching, such that at least k vertices are covered by edges of $\mathcal{E}^*$.
(iii) For a subset $\mathcal{E}^* \subseteq \mathcal{E}$, we define its weight $w(\mathcal{E}^*)$ as the sum of the weights of the edges from $\mathcal{E}^*$.

We consider the following optimization problem.

Problem 1. Min-(b, k)-Matching:
Find a (b, k)-matching with minimum weight, if such a matching exists.

This problem, for certain choices of b and k, specializes to well-known problems in combinatorial optimization:

1. Min-$(1, n)$-Matching is the minimum-weight perfect matching problem in hypergraphs.
2. Min-(m, n)-Matching is the set covering problem in hypergraphs.
3. Min-(m, k)-Matching is the partial set covering (or k-set covering) problem in hypergraphs.

The seed reconstruction problem can be modeled as a minimum-weight perfect matching problem in a 3-uniform hypergraph as follows: let V_1, V_2, V_3 be the seed images on the X-ray photos 1, 2, 3. With $V = V_1 \cup V_2 \cup V_3$ and $\mathcal{E} = V_1 \times V_2 \times V_3$, the hypergraph under consideration is $\mathcal{H}=(V,\mathcal{E})$. Given a weight function $w : \mathcal{E} \to \mathbb{Q} \cap [0,1]$, the seed reconstruction problem is just the problem of finding the minimum-weight perfect matching in $\mathcal{H}$.

2.3 Some probabilistic tools

Throughout this article we consider only finite probability spaces $(\Omega, \mathbb{P})$, where Ω is a finite set and $\mathbb{P}$ is a probability measure with respect to the power set $\mathcal{P}(\Omega)$ as the sigma field. We recall the basic Markov and Chebyshev inequalities.

Theorem 1 (Markov Inequality). *Let $(\Omega, \mathbb{P})$ be a probability space and $X : \Omega \longrightarrow \mathbb{R}^+$ a random variable with expectation $\mathbb{E}(X) < \infty$. Then for any $\lambda \in \mathbb{R}^+$*

$$\mathbb{P}[X \geq \lambda] \leq \frac{\mathbb{E}(X)}{\lambda}.$$

An often sharper bound is the well-known inequality of Chebyshev:

Theorem 2 (Chebyshev Inequality). *Let $(\Omega, \mathbb{P})$ be a probability space and $X : \Omega \longrightarrow \mathbb{R}$ a random variable with finite expectation $\mathbb{E}(X)$ and variance $\mathrm{Var}(X)$. Then for any $\lambda \in \mathbb{R}^+$*

$$\mathbb{P}[|X - \mathbb{E}(X)| \geq \lambda\sqrt{\mathrm{Var}(X)}] \leq \frac{1}{\lambda^2}.$$

For one-sided deviation the following Chebyshev-Cantelli inequality (see [1]) gives better bounds:

Theorem 3. *Let X be a non-negative random variable with finite expectation $\mathbb{E}(X)$ and variance $\mathrm{Var}(X)$. Then for any $a > 0$*

$$\mathbb{P}[X \leq \mathbb{E}(X) - a] \leq \frac{\mathrm{Var}(X)}{\mathrm{Var}(X) + a^2}.$$

The following estimate on the variance of a sum of dependent random variables can be proved as in [1], Corollary 4.3.3.

Let X be the sum of any 0/1 random variables, i.e., $X = X_1 + \ldots + X_n$, and let $p_i = \mathbb{E}(X_i)$ for all $i = 1, \ldots, n$. For a pair $i, j \in \{1, \ldots, n\}$ we write $i \sim j$, if X_i and X_j are dependent. Let Γ be the set of all unordered dependent pairs i, j, i.e., the 2-element sets $\{i, j\}$, and let

$$\gamma = \sum_{\{i,j\} \in \Gamma} \mathbb{E}(X_i X_j).$$

Proposition 1.
$$\text{Var}(X) \le \mathbb{E}(X) + 2\gamma.$$

Proof. We have

$$\text{Var}(X) = \sum_{i=1}^{n} \text{Var}(X_i) + \sum_{i \ne j} \text{Cov}[X_i, X_j], \tag{1}$$

where the second sum is over ordered pairs.

Since $X_i^2 = X_i$, and $\text{Var}(X_i) = \mathbb{E}(X_i^2) - \mathbb{E}(X_i)^2 = \mathbb{E}(X_i)(1 - \mathbb{E}(X_i)) \le \mathbb{E}(X_i)$, (1) gives

$$\text{Var}(X) \le \mathbb{E}(X) + \sum_{i \ne j} \text{Cov}[X_i, X_j]. \tag{2}$$

If $i \nsim j$, then $\text{Cov}[X_i, X_j] = 0$. For $i \sim j$ we have

$$\text{Cov}[X_i, X_j] = \mathbb{E}(X_i X_j) - \mathbb{E}(X_i)\mathbb{E}(X_j) \le \mathbb{E}(X_i X_j), \tag{3}$$

so (3) implies the assertion of the proposition. □

We proceed to the statement of standard large deviation inequalities for a sum of independent random variables.

Let $X_1, \ldots, X_n$ be 0/1 valued mutually independent (briefly: independent) random variables, where

$$\mathbb{P}[X_j = 1] = p_j, \quad \mathbb{P}[X_j = 0] = 1 - p_j$$

for probabilities $p_j \in [0,1]$ for all $1 \le j \le n$. For $1 \le j \le n$ let w_j denote rational weights with

$$0 \le w_j \le 1$$

and let

$$X = \sum_{j=1}^{n} w_j X_j.$$

The sum

$$X = \sum_{j=1}^{n} w_j X_j \text{ with } w_j = 1 \quad \forall \, j \in \{1, \ldots, n\} \tag{4}$$

is the well-known binomially distributed random variable with mean np. The inequalities given below can be found in the books of Alon, Spencer and Erdős [1], Habib, McDiarmid, Ramirez-Alfonsin and Reed [17], and Janson, Łuczak, Ruciński [19].

The following basic large deviation inequality is implicitly given in Chernoff [11] in the binomial case. In explicit form it can be found in Okamoto [23]. Its generalization to arbitrary weight is due to Hoeffding [18].

Theorem 4 ([18]). *Let $\lambda > 0$ and let X be as in (4). Then*

(a) $\mathbb{P}(X > \mathbb{E}(X) + \lambda) \leq e^{-\frac{2\lambda^2}{n}}$.
(b) $\mathbb{P}(X < \mathbb{E}(X) - \lambda) \leq e^{-\frac{2\lambda^2}{n}}$.

In the literature Theorem 4 is well known as the Chernoff bound. For small expectations, i.e., $\mathbb{E}(X) \leq \frac{n}{6}$, the following inequalities due to Angluin and Valiant [5] give better bounds.

Theorem 5. *Let $X_1, \ldots, X_n$ be independent random variables with $0 \leq X_i \leq 1$ and $\mathbb{E}(X_i) = p_i$ for all $i = 1, \ldots, n$. Let $X = \sum_{i=1}^{n} X_i$ and $\mu = \mathbb{E}(X)$. For any $\beta > 0$*

(i) $\mathbb{P}[X \geq (1 + \beta) \cdot \mu] \leq e^{-\frac{\beta^2 \mu}{2(1+\beta/3)}}$.
(ii) $\mathbb{P}[X \leq (1 - \beta) \cdot \mu] \leq e^{-\frac{\beta^2 \mu}{2}}$.

Note that for $0 \leq \beta \leq 3/2$ the bound in (i) is at most $\exp(-\beta^2 \mu/3)$.

We will also need the Landau symbols O, o, Θ and Ω.

Definition 2. *Let $f : \mathbb{N} \to \mathbb{R}_{\geq 0}, g : \mathbb{N} \to \mathbb{R}_{\geq 0}$ be functions. Then*

- $f(n) = O(g(n))$ *if* $\exists \, c_1, c_2 \in \mathbb{R}_{>0}$, *such that*

$$f(n) \leq c_1 g(n) + c_2 \quad \text{for all } n \in \mathbb{N}.$$

- $f(n) = \Omega(g(n))$ *if* $g(n) = O(f(n))$.
- $f(n) = \Theta(g(n))$ *if* $f(n) = O(g(n))$ *and* $f(n) = \Omega(g(n))$.
- $f(n) = o(g(n))$ *if* $\dfrac{f(n)}{g(n)} \overset{n \to \infty}{\longrightarrow} 0$ *(provided that $g(n) \neq 0$ for all n large enough).*

3 Simultaneous matching and covering algorithms

In this section we present a randomized algorithm for the (b, k)-matching problem.

3.1 Randomized algorithms for (b, k)-matching

Let $\mathcal{H} = (V, \mathcal{E}), |V| = n, |\mathcal{E}| = m$ be a hypergraph. We identify the nodes and edges of $\mathcal{H}$ by their indices, so $V = \{1, \ldots, n\}$ and $\mathcal{E} = \{1, \ldots, m\}$. Let $b \geq 1$.

An integer programming formulation of the minimum-weight (b, k)-matching is the following:

Min-(b,k)-ILP $\min \sum_{i=1}^{m} w_i X_i$

$$\sum_{i=1}^{m} a_{ij} X_i \leq b \quad \forall j \in \{1, \dots, n\} \tag{5}$$

$$\sum_{i=1}^{m} a_{ij} X_i \geq Y_j \quad \forall j \in \{1, \dots, n\} \tag{6}$$

$$\sum_{j=1}^{n} Y_j \geq k \tag{7}$$

$$X_i, Y_j \in \{0,1\} \quad \forall i \in \{1, \dots, m\} \, \forall j \in \{1, \dots, n\}. \tag{8}$$

Note that Min-(b,n)-ILP is equivalent to the minimum-weight perfect b-matching problem and Min-(b,k)-ILP is a b-matching problem with a k-partial covering of the vertices.

For the minimum-weight perfect b-matching problems in hypergraphs, where a perfect b-matching exists, for example the 3-uniform hypergraph associated to the seed reconstruction problem, an alternative integer linear programming formulation using local covering conditions is useful.

We add the condition $\sum_{i=1}^{m} a_{ij} X_i \geq \theta$ for some $\theta \in (0,1]$ for all $j \in \{1, \dots, n\}$ to Min-(b,k)-ILP. Then, by integrality all vertices are covered and any feasible solution of such an ILP is a perfect b-matching. For the integer program the additional condition is redundant, but since the LP-relaxation of Min-(b,k)-ILP together with the inequality has a smaller feasible region than the LP-relaxation of Min-(b,k)-ILP, the gap between the integer optimum and the feasible LP-optimum might be smaller as well. This leads to a better "approximation" of the integer optimum by the LP-optimum.

Furthermore, we will see in the theoretical analysis (Section 4) that we can cover significantly more nodes if we add this condition.

Min-(b,k,θ)-ILP $\min \sum_{i=1}^{m} w_i X_i$

$$\sum_{i=1}^{m} a_{ij} X_i \leq b \quad \forall j \in \{1, \dots, n\} \tag{9}$$

$$\sum_{i=1}^{m} a_{ij} X_i \geq Y_j \quad \forall j \in \{1, \dots, n\} \tag{10}$$

$$\sum_{i=1}^{m} a_{ij} X_i \geq \theta \quad \forall j \in \{1, \dots, n\} \tag{11}$$

$$\sum_{j=1}^{n} Y_j \geq k \tag{12}$$

$$X_i, Y_j \in \{0,1\} \quad \forall i \in \{1, \dots, m\} \, \forall j \in \{1, \dots, n\}. \tag{13}$$

We have

Proposition 2. *Let* $\mathcal{H} = (V, \mathcal{E})$ *be a hypergraph with edge weights* $w : \mathcal{E} \to \mathbb{Q}_0^+$. *The integer linear programs* Min-(b, n)-*ILP and* Min-(b, k, θ)-*ILP,* $\theta > 0$, *are equivalent to the minimum-weight perfect b-matching problem in* $\mathcal{H}$.

In the following we need some notations which we fix through the next remark.

Remark 1. Let Min-(b, k, θ)-LP be the linear programming relaxation of Min-(b, k, θ)-ILP. Let (b, k, θ)-ILP be the system of inequalities built by the constraints (9) - (13) of Min-(b, k, θ)-ILP, and let (b, k, θ)-LP be the LP-relaxation of (b, k, θ)-ILP, where $X_i \in [0, 1] \cap \mathbb{Q}$ and $Y_j \in \mathbb{Q}_0^+$ for all i, j.

3.2 The randomized algorithm

Before we state the randomized algorithm, we have to ensure whether or not a Min-(b, k, θ)-matching exists. For a given b, a choice of $k = 0$ and $\theta = 0$ always makes the problem feasible. However, for some k and θ there might be no solution. Then we would like to find the maximum k such that a solution exists, given b and θ. Actually, for the integer programs we have to distinguish only between the cases $\theta = 0$ and $\theta > 0$ (which is the perfect b-matching problem).

Algorithm LP-Search(θ)

Input: $\theta \geq 0$.

1) Test the solvability of $(b, 0, \theta)$-LP. If it is not solvable, return "$(b, 0, \theta)$-LP is not feasible." Otherwise set $k := 1$ and go to 2.
2) a) Test solvability of (b, k, θ)-LP and $(b, k + 1, \theta)$-LP.
   b) If both are solvable, set $k := k + 2$ and go to 2a. If (b, k, θ)-LP is solvable, but $(b, k + 1, \theta)$-LP is not solvable, return k.   □

If $(b, 0, \theta)$-LP is solvable, we define

$$k^* := \max \{k \in \mathbb{N} ; k \leq n ; (b, k, \theta)\text{-}LP \text{ has a solution}\}.$$

Obviously we have

Proposition 3. *The algorithm* LP-Search (θ) *either outputs "$(b, 0, \theta)$-LP is not feasible" or solving at most n LPs, it returns* k^*.

It is clear that the number of iterations can be dropped to at most $\lceil \log(n) \rceil$ using binary search.

In the following we work with a $k \in \mathbb{N}$, returned by the algorithm LP-Search(θ), if it exists. The randomized rounding algorithm for the Min-(b, k, θ)-matching problem is the following:

ALGORITHM MIN-(b, k, θ)-RR

1. Solve the LP-relaxation Min-(b, k, θ)-ILP optimally, with solutions $x^* = (x_1^*, \ldots, x_m^*)$ and $y^* = (y_1^*, \ldots, y_n^*)$. Let $OPT^* = \sum_{i=1}^{m} w_i x_i^*$.
2. *Randomized Rounding*: Choose $\delta \in (0, 1]$. For $i = 1, \ldots, m$, independently set the 0/1 random variable X_i to 1 with probability δx_i^* and to 0 with probability $1 - \delta x_i^*$. So
   $\Pr[X_i = 1] = \delta x_i^*$ and $\Pr[X_i = 0] = 1 - \delta x_i^*$, $\forall i \in \{1, \ldots, m\}$.
3. Output $X_1, \ldots, X_m$, the set of hyperedges $\mathcal{M}' = \{i \in \mathcal{E}; x_i = 1\}$, and its weight $w(\mathcal{M}')$. □

One can combine the algorithm Min-(b, k, θ)-RR with a greedy approach in order to get a feasible b-matching:

ALGORITHM MIN-(b, k, θ)-ROUND

1) Apply the algorithm MIN-(b, k, θ)-RR and output a set of hyperedges $\mathcal{M}'$.
2) List the nodes in a randomized order. Passing through this list and arriving at a node for which the b-matching condition is violated, we enforce the b-matching condition at this node by removing incident edges from $\mathcal{M}'$ with highest weights.
3) Output is the so obtained set $\mathcal{M} \subseteq \mathcal{M}'$. □

Variants of this algorithm are possible, for example, one can remove edges incident in many nodes, etc..

4 Main results and proofs

4.1 The main results

We present an analysis of the algorithm MIN-(b, k, θ)-RR. Our most general result is the following theorem. C_1 and C_2 are positive constants depending only on l, δ, and θ. They will specified more precisely later.

Theorem 6. *Let $\delta \in (0, 1)$ and $OPT^* \geq \frac{2}{3} \ln(4)(1 + 2\delta)(1 - \delta)^{-2}$. For $\lambda = \sqrt{\frac{m}{2} \ln(4n)}$ we have:*

(a) *Let $\Delta \leq c_1 \cdot \frac{k}{b}$. For $\theta = 0$, the algorithm MIN-(b, k, θ)-RR returns a $(\delta b + \lambda)$-matching $\mathcal{M}'$ in $\mathcal{H}$ of weight $w(\mathcal{M}') \leq OPT^*$ which covers at least*

$$\frac{k}{b}(1 - e^{-\delta b}) \left(1 - \sqrt{\frac{3b(\Delta(l - 1) + 3)}{2k(1 - e^{-\delta b})}}\right) \tag{14}$$

nodes of $\mathcal{H}$ with a probability of at least $1/4$.

(b) *Let* $\Delta \leq c_2 \cdot n$. *For* $\theta > 0$ *the algorithm* MIN-(b, k, θ)-RR *returns a* $(\delta b + \lambda)$-*matching* $\mathcal{M}'$ *in* $\mathcal{H}$ *of weight* $w(\mathcal{M}') \leq OPT^*$ *which covers at least*

$$0.632\delta\theta n \left(1 - \sqrt{\frac{2.38(\Delta(l-1)+3)}{\delta\theta n}}\right) \tag{15}$$

nodes of $\mathcal{H}$ *with a probability of at least* $1/4$.

For special b, we have a stronger result.

Theorem 7. *Let* $\delta \in (0,1)$. *Assume that*

 i) $b \geq \frac{2}{3}\ln(4n)(1+2\delta)(1-\delta)^{-2}$.
 ii) $OPT^* \geq \frac{2}{3}\ln(4)(1+2\delta)(1-\delta)^{-2}$.

(a) *Let* $\Delta \leq c_1 \cdot \frac{k}{b}$. *For* $\theta = 0$, *the algorithm* MIN-(b, k, θ)-RR *returns a* b-*matching* $\mathcal{M}'$ *in* $\mathcal{H}$ *of weight* $w(\mathcal{M}') \leq OPT^*$ *which covers at least*

$$\frac{k}{b}(1 - e^{-\delta b})\left(1 - \sqrt{\frac{3b(\Delta(l-1)+3)}{2k(1-e^{-\delta b})}}\right)$$

nodes of $\mathcal{H}$ *with a probability of at least* $1/4$.
(b) *Let* $\Delta \leq c_2 \cdot n$. *For* $\theta > 0$ *the algorithm* MIN-(b, k, θ)-RR *returns a* b-*matching* $\mathcal{M}'$ *in* $\mathcal{H}$ *of weight* $w(\mathcal{M}') \leq OPT^*$ *which covers at least*

$$0.632\delta\theta n \left(1 - \sqrt{\frac{2.38(\Delta(l-1)+3)}{\delta\theta n}}\right)$$

nodes of $\mathcal{H}$ *with a probability of at least* $1/4$.

Remark 2. In Theorem 7 (a), for fixed δ, we have $b = \Omega(\ln(n))$. For $b = \Theta(\ln(n))$, and $k = \Omega(n)$ and $\Delta \leq c_1 \cdot \frac{k}{b}$, the number of covered nodes is at least

$$\Omega\left(\frac{n}{\ln(n)}(1-o(1))\right). \tag{16}$$

In this case we have an approximation of the maximum number of covered nodes k up to a factor of $1/\ln(n)$. From the techniques applied so far it is not clear whether the coverage can be improved towards $\Omega(k)$.

4.2 Proofs

We will first prove Theorem 7 and then 6. We start with a technical lemma.

Lemma 1. *Let* $X_1, \ldots, X_m$ *be independent* $0/1$ *random variables with* $\mathbb{E}(X_i) = p_i \ \forall i = 1, \ldots, m$. *For* $w_i \in [0, 1], i = 1, \ldots, n, w(X) := \sum_{i=1}^{m} w_i X_i$. *Let* $z \geq 0$ *be an upper bound on* $\mathbb{E}(w(X))$, *i.e.,* $\mathbb{E}(w(X)) \leq z$. *Then*

i) $\mathbb{P}[w(X) \geq z(1 + \beta)] \leq e^{-\frac{\beta^2 z}{2(1+\beta/3)}}$ *for any* $\beta > 0$.

ii) $\mathbb{P}[w(X) \geq z(1 + \beta)] \leq e^{-\frac{\beta^2 z}{3}}$ *for* $0 \leq \beta \leq 1$.

Proof. Let $z' := \lfloor z - \mathbb{E}(w(X)) \rfloor, p = z - \mathbb{E}(w(X)) - z'$, and let $Y_0, Y_1, \ldots, Y_{z'}$ be independent $0/1$ random variables with $\mathbb{E}(Y_0) = p$ and $Y_j = 1 \ \forall j \geq 1$. The random variable $X' := w(X) + Y_0 + Y_1 + \ldots + Y_{z'}$ satisfies $\mathbb{E}(X') = z$ and $X' \geq w(X)$ and we may apply the Angluin-Valiant inequality (Theorem 5) to it:

i) For any $\beta > 0$ we have

$$\mathbb{P}[w(X) \geq z(1 + \beta)] \leq \mathbb{P}[X' \geq z(1 + \beta)] \leq e^{-\frac{\beta^2 z}{2(1+\beta/3)}}.$$

ii) For $0 \leq \beta \leq 1$ it is easy to see that $e^{-\frac{\beta^2 z}{2(1+\beta/3)}} \leq e^{-\frac{\beta^2 z}{3}}$. □

Let $X_1, \ldots, X_m$ and $\mathcal{M}'$ be the output of the algorithm MIN-(b, k, θ)-RR. Further let OPT and OPT^* be the integer respectively LP-optima for Min-(b, k, θ)-ILP.

Lemma 2. *Suppose that* $\delta \in (0, 1)$ *and* $b \geq \frac{2}{3} \ln(4n)(1 + 2\delta)(1 - \delta)^{-2}$. *Then*

$$\mathbb{P}\left[\exists j \in V : \sum_{i=1}^{m} a_{ij} X_i \geq b\right] \leq \frac{1}{4}.$$

Proof. First we compute the expectation

$$\mathbb{E}\left(\sum_{i=1}^{m} a_{ij} X_i\right) = \sum_{i=1}^{m} a_{ij} \mathbb{E}(X_i) = \sum_{i=1}^{m} a_{ij} \delta x_i^* = \delta \cdot \sum_{i=1}^{m} a_{ij} x_i^* \leq \delta b. \quad (17)$$

Set $\beta := \frac{1}{\delta} - 1$. With Lemma 1 we get:

$$\mathbb{P}\left[\sum_{i=1}^{m} a_{ij} X_i \geq b\right] = \mathbb{P}\left[\sum_{i=1}^{m} a_{ij} X_i \geq (1 + \beta)\delta b\right]$$

$$\leq \exp\left(\frac{-\beta^2 \delta b}{2(1 + \beta/3)}\right)$$

$$= \exp\left(-\frac{3}{2} \cdot \frac{(1 - \delta)^2}{1 + 2\delta} \cdot b\right)$$

$$\leq \frac{1}{4n} \quad \text{(using the assumption on } b\text{)}.$$

So

$$\mathbb{P}\left[\exists j \in V : \sum_{i=1}^{m} a_{ij} X_i \geq b\right] \leq \sum_{j=1}^{n} \mathbb{P}\left[\sum_{i=1}^{m} a_{ij} X_i \geq b\right] \leq n \cdot \left(\frac{1}{4n}\right) = \frac{1}{4}. \quad □$$

Lemma 3. *Suppose that $\delta \in (0,1)$ and $OPT^* \geq \frac{2}{3}\ln(4)(1+2\delta)(1-\delta)^{-2}$. Then*

$$\mathbb{P}\left[\sum_{i=1}^{m} w_i X_i \geq OPT^*\right] \leq \frac{1}{4}.$$

Proof. We have

$$\mathbb{E}\left(\sum_{i=1}^{m} w_i X_i\right) = \sum_{i=1}^{m} w_i \mathbb{E}(X_i) = \sum_{i=1}^{m} w_i \delta x_i^* = \delta \cdot \sum_{i=1}^{m} w_i x_i^* = \delta \cdot OPT^*. \quad (18)$$

Choose $\beta = \frac{1}{\delta} - 1$. Then

$$\mathbb{P}\left[\sum_{i=1}^{m} w_i X_i \geq OPT^*\right] = \mathbb{P}\left[\sum_{i=1}^{m} w_i X_i \geq \delta(1+\beta)\,OPT^*\right]$$

$$= \mathbb{P}\left[\sum_{i=1}^{m} w_i X_i \geq \mathbb{E}\left(\sum_{i=1}^{m} w_i X_i\right)(1+\beta)\right]$$

$$\leq \exp\left(\frac{-\beta^2 \mathbb{E}(\sum_{i=1}^{m} w_i X_i)}{2(1+\beta/3)}\right) \quad \text{(Theorem 5(i))}$$

$$= \exp\left(\frac{-\beta^2\, \delta\, OPT^*}{2(1+\beta/3)}\right)$$

$$\leq \frac{1}{4}$$

where the last inequality follows from the assumption on OPT^*.   □

We now come to a key lemma, which controls the covering quality of the randomized algorithm.

Let $Y_j := \sum_{i=1}^{m} a_{ij} X_i$ for all j and $Y := \sum_{j=1}^{n} Y_j$.

Lemma 4. *For any $\delta \in (0,1]$,*

i) $\mathbb{E}(Y) \geq n - \sum_{j=1}^{n} e^{-\delta \sum_{i=1}^{m} a_{ij} x_i^*}$,

ii) *If $\theta > 0$, then $\mathbb{E}(Y) \geq n(1-e^{-\delta\theta}) \geq 0.632\delta\theta n$,*

iii) *For Min-(b,k,θ)-RR with $\theta = 0$ we have $\mathbb{E}(Y) \geq \frac{k}{b}(1-e^{-\delta b})$.*

Proof. i) Define $\mathcal{E}_j := \{E \in \mathcal{E}; j \in E\}$. We have

$$\mathbb{E}(Y) = \mathbb{E}\left(\sum_{j=1}^{n} Y_j\right) = \sum_{j=1}^{n} \mathbb{E}(Y_j) = \sum_{j=1}^{n} \mathbb{P}[Y_j = 1]$$

$$= \sum_{j=1}^{n}(1 - \mathbb{P}[Y_j = 0]) = n - \sum_{j=1}^{n} \mathbb{P}[Y_j = 0]. \quad (19)$$

Now

$$\mathbb{P}[Y_j = 0] = \mathbb{P}\left[\sum_{i=1}^{m} a_{ij}X_i = 0\right]$$
$$= \mathbb{P}[(a_{1j}X_1 = 0) \wedge \ldots \wedge (a_{mj}X_m = 0)]$$
$$= \prod_{i=1}^{m} \mathbb{P}[a_{ij}X_i = 0]$$
$$= \prod_{i \in \mathcal{E}_j} \mathbb{P}[X_i = 0]$$
$$= \prod_{i \in \mathcal{E}_j} (1 - \delta x_i^*). \tag{20}$$

For $u \in \mathbb{R}$ we have the inequality $1 - u \le e^{-u}$. Thus

$$\prod_{i \in \mathcal{E}_j} (1 - \delta x_i^*) \le \prod_{i \in \mathcal{E}_j} e^{-\delta x_i^*} = e^{-\delta \cdot \sum_{i=1}^{m} a_{ij}x_i^*}. \tag{21}$$

Hence, with (19),(20) and (21)

$$\mathbb{E}(Y) \ge n - \sum_{j=1}^{n} e^{-\delta \cdot \sum_{i=1}^{m} a_{ij}x_i^*}. \tag{22}$$

ii) Since $\sum_{i=1}^{m} a_{ij}x_i^* \ge \theta$ for all $j \in \{1, \ldots, n\}$, the first inequality immediately follows from (i). For the second inequality, observe that for $x \in [0,1], e^{-x} \le 1 - x + x/e$. This is true, because the linear function $1 - x + x/e$ is an upper bound for the convex function e^{-x} in $[0,1]$. So $\mathbb{E}(Y) \ge (1 - e^{-\delta\theta})n \ge (1 - 1/e)\delta\theta n \ge 0.632\delta\theta n$.

iii) Since e^{-x} is convex, the linear function $1 - x(\delta b)^{-1} + xe^{-\delta b}(\delta b)^{-1}$ is an upper bound for e^{-x} in $[0, \delta b]$. With (22) we get

$$\mathbb{E}(Y) \ge n - n + (1 - e^{-\delta b})\delta(\delta b)^{-1} \underbrace{\sum_{j=1}^{n} \sum_{i=1}^{m} a_{ij}x_i^*}_{\ge k} \ge (1 - e^{-\delta b}) \cdot \frac{k}{b}. \qquad \Box$$

An upper bound for the variance of Y can be computed directly, via covariance and dependent pairs:

Lemma 5. *Let Δ be the maximum vertex degree of $\mathcal{H}$ and let l be the maximum cardinality of a hyperedge. Then*

$$\mathrm{Var}(Y) \le \frac{1}{2} \cdot (\Delta(l - 1) + 3)\mathbb{E}(Y).$$

Proof. By Proposition 1

$$\text{Var}(Y) \le \mathbb{E}(Y) + 2\gamma \tag{23}$$

where γ is the sum of $\mathbb{E}(Y_i Y_j)$ of all unordered dependent pairs i, j. Since the Y_is are $0/1$ random variables, we have for pairs $\{i, j\}$ with $i \sim j$

$$
\begin{aligned}
\mathbb{E}(Y_i Y_j) &= \mathbb{P}[(Y_i = 1) \wedge (Y_j = 1)] \\
&\le \min(\mathbb{P}[Y_i = 1], \mathbb{P}[Y_j = 1]) \\
&\le \frac{1}{2}(\mathbb{P}[Y_i = 1] + \mathbb{P}[Y_j = 1]) \\
&= \frac{1}{2}(\mathbb{E}(Y_i) + \mathbb{E}(Y_j)).
\end{aligned}
$$

Hence

$$
\begin{aligned}
\gamma &= \sum_{\{i,j\} \in \Gamma} \mathbb{E}(Y_i Y_j) \le \frac{1}{2} \sum_{\{i,j\} \in \Gamma} (\mathbb{E}(Y_i) + \mathbb{E}(Y_j)) \\
&\le \frac{1}{4} \sum_{i=1}^{n} \left(\mathbb{E}(Y_i) + \sum_{j \sim i} \mathbb{E}(Y_j) \right) = \frac{1}{4} \mathbb{E}(Y) + \frac{1}{4} \sum_{i=1}^{n} \sum_{j \sim i} \mathbb{E}(Y_j) \\
&\le \frac{1}{4} \mathbb{E}(Y) + \frac{1}{4} \sum_{i=1}^{n} \mathbb{E}(Y_i) \Delta(l-1) = \frac{1}{4} \mathbb{E}(Y) + \frac{1}{4} \Delta(l-1) \mathbb{E}(Y) \\
&= \frac{1}{4}(\Delta(l-1)+1) \mathbb{E}(Y),
\end{aligned}
$$

and (23) concludes the proof.   □

Let c_1 and c_2 be positive constants depending only on $l, \delta,$ and θ such that for $\Delta \le c_1 \cdot \frac{k}{b}$ respectively $\Delta \le c_2 \cdot n$ we have

$$\sqrt{\frac{3b(\Delta(l-1)+3)}{2k(1-e^{-\delta b})}} < 1 \text{ respectively } \sqrt{\frac{2.38(\Delta(l-1)+3)}{\delta\theta n}} < 1. \tag{24}$$

Note that in the following we assume $l, \delta,$ and θ to be constants.

Lemma 6.

i) *For* $a := \sqrt{\frac{3}{2}(\Delta(l-1)+3)\mathbb{E}(Y)}: \quad \mathbb{P}[Y \le \mathbb{E}(Y) - a] \le \frac{1}{4}.$

ii) *Let* $\Delta \le c_1 \cdot \frac{k}{b}.$ *Then*

$$\mathbb{E}(Y) - a \ge \frac{k}{b}(1 - e^{-\delta b}) \left(1 - \sqrt{\frac{3b(\Delta(l-1)+3)}{2k(1-e^{-\delta b})}} \right) \quad \text{if} \quad \theta = 0.$$

iii) *Let* $\Delta \leq c_2 \cdot n$. *Then*

$$\mathbb{E}(Y) - a \geq 0.632\delta\theta n \left(1 - \sqrt{\frac{2.38(\Delta(l-1)+3)}{\delta\theta n}}\right) \quad \text{if} \quad \theta > 0.$$

Proof. i) With the Chebyshev-Cantelli inequality (Theorem 3) we have

$$\mathbb{P}[Y \leq \mathbb{E}(Y) - a] \leq \frac{\text{Var}(Y)}{\text{Var}(Y) + a^2} = \frac{1}{1 + \frac{a^2}{\text{Var}(Y)}}$$

$$\leq \frac{1}{1 + \frac{a^2}{0.5(\Delta(l-1)+3)\mathbb{E}(Y)}} \quad \text{(Lemma 5)}$$

$$= \frac{1}{1 + \frac{1.5(\Delta(l-1)+3)\mathbb{E}(Y)}{0.5(\Delta(l-1)+3)\mathbb{E}(Y)}} = \frac{1}{4}.$$

ii) and iii):

$$\mathbb{E}(Y) - a = \mathbb{E}(Y)\left(1 - \frac{\sqrt{\frac{3}{2}(\Delta(l-1)+3)\mathbb{E}(Y)}}{\mathbb{E}(Y)}\right) \tag{25}$$

$$= \mathbb{E}(Y)\left(1 - \frac{\sqrt{3(\Delta(l-1)+3)}}{\sqrt{2\mathbb{E}(Y)}}\right) \tag{26}$$

$$\geq \begin{cases} \frac{k}{b}(1 - e^{-\delta b})\left(1 - \sqrt{\frac{3b(\Delta(l-1)+3)}{2k(1-e^{-\delta b})}}\right) & \text{if} \quad \theta = 0, \\ 0.632\delta\theta n\left(1 - \sqrt{\frac{2.38(\Delta(l-1)+3)}{\delta\theta n}}\right) & \text{if} \quad \theta > 0. \end{cases} \tag{27}$$

Note that to the upper bound condition for Δ, the lower bounds in (27) are positive. □

Proof (Theorem 7). Lemma 2, 3 and 6 imply Theorem 7. □

This theorem holds only for $b = \Omega(\ln(n))$. In the rest of this section we give an analysis also for the case of arbitrary b, losing a certain amount of feasibility.

Lemma 7. *Let* $\delta > 0$, $\mu_j = \mathbb{E}(\sum_{i=1}^m a_{ij}X_i)$ *for all* j, *and* $\lambda = \sqrt{\frac{m}{2}\ln(4n)}$. *Then*

$$\mathbb{P}\left[\exists j : \sum_{i=1}^m a_{ij}X_i > \delta b + \lambda\right] \leq \frac{1}{4}.$$

Proof. As in (17), $\mu_j = \mathbb{E}(\sum_{i=1}^{m} a_{ij} X_i) \leq \delta b$ for all j. With the Chernoff-Hoeffding bound (Theorem 4)

$$\mathbb{P}\left[\sum_{i=1}^{m} a_{ij} X_i > \delta b + \lambda\right] \leq \mathbb{P}\left[\sum_{i=1}^{m} a_{ij} X_i > \mu_j + \lambda\right]$$

$$\leq \exp\left(\frac{-2\lambda^2}{m}\right) = \exp\left(-\ln(4n)\right) = \frac{1}{4n}.$$

So,

$$\mathbb{P}\left[\exists\, j \in V : \sum_{i=1}^{m} a_{ij} X_i > \delta b + \lambda\right]$$

$$\leq \sum_{j=1}^{n} \mathbb{P}\left[\sum_{i=1}^{m} a_{ij} X_i > \delta b + \lambda\right] \leq n \cdot \left(\frac{1}{4n}\right) = \frac{1}{4}. \quad \square$$

Proof (Theorem 6). Lemma 3, 6 and 7 imply Theorem 6. $\square$

5 Experimental results

5.1 Implementation

We run the algorithm MIN-(b, k, θ)-ROUND for different values of b, k, and θ in a C^{++}-implementation.

Recall that the algorithm MIN-(b, k, θ)-ROUND has 3 steps:

1. It solves the linear program and delivers a fractional solution,
2. applies randomized rounding on the fractional solution and delivers an integer solution, which we call *primary solution,*
3. removes edges from the primary solution.

In the primary solution the nodes might be covered by more than b edges. The superfluous edges are removed in step 3. Edges are removed in a randomized greedy approach. The nodes are chosen in a randomized order and if the considered node is covered by more than one edge, the ones with the greatest cost are removed. In the following tables we use 100 runs of the randomized rounding algorithm. As the final solution, we choose the one with the fewest number of uncovered nodes. (If this choice is not unique, we pick one with the smallest cost.) The LPs are solved with a simplex-method with the CLP-solver from the free COIN-OR library [21].

The columns in the tables in Sections 5.2 and 5.3 are organized as follows:

1: represents patient data
   (Patients 1-5 are real patient data, whereas Patient 6 is a phantom.)
2: represents number of seeds to be matched
3: represents the cost of the LP-solution
4: represents the cost of the matching returned by the algorithm
5: represents the running time in CPU seconds of the program
6: represents number of unmatched seeds

5.2 Results for the algorithm MIN-(b, k, θ)-ROUND

Table 1. $b = 1.20$, $k = 0.90 \cdot n$, $\theta = 0.00$.

Patient	Seeds	LP-OPT	Cost	Time	Unmatched
1	67	54.31	48.30	14.23	12
2	67	77.03	66.02	14.61	14
3	31	17.08	16.62	1.01	4
4	22	17.96	17.18	0.32	3
5	43	72.39	53.43	3.40	13
6	25	5.30	4.42	0.50	6

Table 2. $b = 1.20$, $k = 1.00 \cdot n$, $\theta = 0.00$.

Patient	Seeds	LP-OPT	Cost	Time	Unmatched
1	67	67.77	58.20	14.73	7
2	67	93.32	78.22	14.54	9
3	31	21.18	19.44	1.02	2
4	22	21.94	19.24	0.33	2
5	43	91.34	55.33	3.59	14
6	25	6.51	5.44	0.51	4

Table 3. $b = 1.10$, $k = 0.90 \cdot n$, $\theta = 0.00$.

Patient	Seeds	LP-OPT	Cost	Time	Unmatched
1	67	56.40	54.11	14.23	9
2	67	80.20	75.61	14.60	10
3	31	17.41	16.62	1.00	4
4	22	18.20	17.18	0.32	3
5	43	79.77	63.41	3.61	11
6	25	5.71	4.91	0.52	5

Table 4. $b = 1.10$, $k = 1.00 \cdot n$, $\theta = 0.00$.

Patient	Seeds	LP-OPT	Cost	Time	Unmatched
1	67	71.59	63.12	15.23	5
2	67	98.13	88.89	15.52	5
3	31	21.84	20.97	1.01	1
4	22	22.78	21.50	0.34	1
5	43	103.85	68.53	4.10	12
6	25	7.22	6.69	0.51	2

Table 5. $b = 1.00$, $k = 0.90 \cdot n$, $\theta = 0.00$.

Patient	Seeds	LP-OPT	Cost	Time	Unmatched
1	67	58.91	60.56	14.81	6
2	67	84.17	86.11	14.34	6
3	31	17.80	17.94	1.01	3
4	22	18.83	19.24	0.34	2
5	43	91.67	66.53	3.95	13
6	25	6.37	6.69	0.51	2

Table 6. $b = 1.00$, $k = 1.00 \cdot n$, $\theta = 0.00$.

Patient	Seeds	LP-OPT	Cost	Time	Unmatched
1	67	80.60	80.60	15.59	0
2	67	170.27	119.53	33.48	8
3	31	22.58	22.58	1.01	0
4	22	23.82	23.82	0.33	0
5	43	199.65	199.65	7.40	0
6	25	8.85	8.85	0.54	0

5.3 Results for the algorithm MIN-(b, k, θ)-ROUND with $\theta > 0$

Table 7. $b = 1.20$, $k = 0.90 \cdot n$, $\theta = 0.20$.

Patient	Seeds	LP-OPT	Cost	Time	Unmatched
1	67	55.27	55.10	14.26	9
2	67	80.33	74.11	14.34	11
3	31	17.29	18.57	1.01	3
4	22	18.17	19.24	0.33	2
5	43	74.77	51.90	3.49	14
6	25	5.51	3.99	0.52	7

Table 8. $b = 1.20$, $k = 1.00 \cdot n$, $\theta = 0.20$.

Patient	Seeds	LP-OPT	Cost	Time	Unmatched
1	67	68.25	60.76	14.31	6
2	67	96.20	78.11	14.73	9
3	31	21.22	20.97	1.01	1
4	22	21.94	19.24	0.33	2
5	43	92.77	55.19	3.70	13
6	25	6.66	4.91	0.52	5

Table 9. $b = 1.10$, $k = 0.90 \cdot n$, $\theta = 0.20$.

Patient	Seeds	LP-OPT	Cost	Time	Unmatched
1	67	57.41	57.01	14.17	8
2	67	83.51	75.54	14.48	11
3	31	17.61	19.73	1.01	2
4	22	18.45	19.24	0.32	2
5	43	81.39	55.20	3.64	13
6	25	5.89	4.48	0.51	6

Table 10. $b = 1.10$, $k = 1.00 \cdot n$, $\theta = 0.20$.

Patient	Seeds	LP-OPT	Cost	Time	Unmatched
1	67	71.79	63.12	14.88	5
2	67	100.78	93.04	15.32	4
3	31	21.85	22.58	1.02	0
4	22	22.79	23.82	0.33	0
5	43	104.57	72.66	3.89	13
6	25	7.32	6.69	0.52	2

Table 11. $b = 1.00$, $k = 0.90 \cdot n$, $\theta = 0.20$.

Patient	Seeds	LP-OPT	Cost	Time	Unmatched
1	67	59.93	63.64	14.19	5
2	67	87.51	87.97	14.43	6
3	31	17.94	20.97	1.02	1
4	22	18.92	21.56	0.33	1
5	43	92.40	58.17	3.91	15
6	25	6.48	6.69	0.52	2

Table 12. $b = 1.00$, $k = 1.00 \cdot n$, $\theta = 0.20$.

Patient	Seeds	LP-OPT	Cost	Time	Unmatched
1	67	80.60	80.60	15.92	0
2	67	170.27	115.10	31.82	8
3	31	22.58	22.58	1.01	0
4	22	23.82	23.82	0.33	0
5	43	199.65	199.65	7.77	0
6	25	8.85	8.85	0.52	0

Table 13. $b = 1.20$, $k = 0.90 \cdot n$, $\theta = 1.00$.

Patient	Seeds	LP-OPT	Cost	Time	Unmatched
1	67	79.80	76.20	14.49	1
2	67	122.16	111.16	15.96	2
3	31	22.58	22.58	1.01	0
4	22	23.78	23.82	0.33	0
5	43	129.47	77.03	4.58	12
6	25	8.80		0.52	0

Table 14. $b = 1.20$, $k = 1.00 \cdot n$, $\theta = 1.00$.

Patient	Seeds	LP-OPT	Cost	Time	Unmatched
1	67	79.80	76.20	14.83	1
2	67	122.16	111.16	16.34	2
3	31	22.58	22.58	1.04	0
4	22	23.78	23.82	0.34	0
5	43	129.47	77.62	4.54	12
6	25	8.80	8.85	0.53	0

Table 15. $b = 1.10$, $k = 0.90 \cdot n$, $\theta = 1.00$.

Patient	Seeds	LP-OPT	Cost	Time	Unmatched
1	67	80.20	80.60	14.49	0
2	67	125.93	108.72	16.90	3
3	31	22.58	22.58	1.01	0
4	22	23.80	23.82	0.34	0
5	43	142.54	92.19	5.09	11
6	25	8.83	8.85	0.50	0

Table 16. $b = 1.10$, $k = 1.00 \cdot n$, $\theta = 1.00$.

Patient	Seeds	LP-OPT	Cost	Time	Unmatched
1	67	80.20	80.60	15.37	0
2	67	125.93	108.72	17.42	3
3	31	22.58	22.58	1.04	0
4	22	23.80	23.82	0.33	0
5	43	142.54	90.05	4.98	11
6	25	8.83	8.85	0.52	0

Table 17. $b = 1.00$, $k = 0.90 \cdot n$, $\theta = 1.00$.

Patient	Seeds	LP-OPT	Cost	Time	Unmatched
1	67	80.60	80.60	14.74	0
2	67	170.27	111.85	25.48	8
3	31	22.58	22.58	1.01	0
4	22	23.82	23.82	0.33	0
5	43	199.65	199.65	6.50	0
6	25	8.85	8.85	0.52	0

Table 18. $b = 1.00$, $k = 1.00 \cdot n$, $\theta = 1.00$.

Patient	Seeds	LP-OPT	Cost	Time	Unmatched
1	67	80.60	80.60	14.24	0
2	67	170.27	113.91	25.65	7
3	31	22.58	22.58	0.99	0
4	22	23.82	23.82	0.32	0
5	43	199.65	199.65	6.48	0
6	25	8.85	8.85	0.51	0

5.4 Discussion — implementation *vs.* theory

With the algorithm MIN-(b, k, θ)-ROUND for $\theta = 0$, we get optimal results (except Patient 2) if the constraints are most restrictive: $b = 1.00$, $k = 1.00 \cdot n$, see Table 6. With the algorithm MIN-(b, k, θ)-ROUND for $\theta > 0$, the same observation holds: optimal results (except Patient 2) are achieved with the most restrictive constraints: $b = 1.00$, $k = 1.00 \cdot n$, $\theta = 0.2$ (Table 12) and $b = 1.00$, $k = 1.00 \cdot n$, $\theta = 1.00$ (Table 18). Obviously, a high θ can compensate for a low k, and vice versa (see Table 5 in comparison to 17, and 5 in comparison to 6).

This clearly shows that the practical results for the instances are much better than the analysis of Section 4 indicates. However, to close the gap between theory and practice seems to be a challenging problem in the area of randomized algorithms, where the so far developed probabilistic tools seem to be insufficient.

The non-optimal results for Patient 2 could be explained by the bad image quality of the X-rays and movement of the patient in the time between taking two different X-rays.

Since it is important to find the correct matching of the seeds and not just any minimum-weight perfect matching, the question of whether this is the right matching is legitimate. This is difficult to prove, but results with help of a graphical 3D-program seem to be promising: we take the proposed seed positions in 3D and produce pictures, showing how the seeds would lie on the X-rays if these were the real positions. A comparison between the pictures and the real X-rays shows that the positions agree.

This observation is supported by the results for the phantom (Patient 6), where we know the seed positions, and where the algorithm returns the optimal solution, see, e.g., Table 18.

The running times of our algorithm are of the same order of magnitude as those of the commercial software VariSeed® presently used at the Clinic of Radiotherapy. These range between 4 and 20 seconds for instances with

43 to 82 seeds respectively. However — due to technical and licensing issues — we had to measure these times on a different computer (different CPU and operating system, but approximately the same frequency) than the one where the tests for our algorithm were performed, and we also had no exact method of measurement available (just a stopwatch). As we are dealing with an off-line application, a few seconds in running time are unimportant. Also our implementation can likely be improved (especially the part for reading in the large instance files) to gain even a few seconds in running time and possibly outperform the commercial software with respect to running time.

Our main advantage, however, lies in the quality of the solution delivered. Our algorithm also delivered the correct solution in certain cases where the commercial one failed. As shown by Siebert et al. [25], VariSeed® (versions 6.7/7.1) can compute wrong 3D seed distributions if seeds are arranged in certain ways, and these errors cannot be explained by the ambiguities inherent to the three-film technique. Our algorithm, however, performs well on the phantom instance studied in [25] (as well as on the tested patient data, except for Patient 2, which had a poor image quality). As a consequence, the immigration of our algorithm in the brachytherapy planning process at the Clinic of Radiotherapy in Kiel is planned.

6 Open problems

Most interesting are the following problems, which we leave open but would like to discuss in future work.

1. At the moment, we can analyze the randomized rounding algorithm, but we are not able to analyze the repairing step of the algorithm MIN-(b, k, θ)-ROUND. But this of course is a major challenge for future work.
2. Can the coverage of $\Omega\left(\frac{k}{b}\right)$ in Theorem 7 be improved towards $\Omega(k)$?
3. Can the b-matching lower bound assumption $b = \Omega(\ln(n))$ in Theorem 7 be dropped towards $b = O(1)$?
4. What is the approximation complexity of the minimum-weight perfect matching problem in hypergraphs? Is there a complexity-theoretic threshold?

References

1. N. Alon, J. Spencer, and P. Erdős. *The Probabilistic Method.* John Wiley & Sons, Inc., 1992.
2. M. D. Altschuler, R. D. Epperson, and P. A. Findlay. Rapid, accurate, three-dimensional location of multiple seeds in implant radiotherapy treatment planning. *Physics in Medicine and Biology*, 28:1305–1318, 1983.

3. H. I. Amols, G. N. Cohen, D. A. Todor, and M. Zaider. Operator-free, film-based 3D seed reconstruction in brachytherapy. *Physics in Medicine and Biology*, 47:2031–2048, 2002.

4. H. I. Amols and I. I. Rosen. A three-film technique for reconstruction of radioactive seed implants. *Medical Physics*, 8:210–214, 1981.

5. D. Angluin and L. G. Valiant. Fast probabilistic algorithms for Hamiltonian circuits and matchings. *Journal of Computer and System Sciences*, 18:155–193, 1979.

6. D. Ash, J. Battermann, L. Blank, A. Flynn, T. de Reijke, and P. Lavagnini. ESTRO/EAU/EORTC recommendations on permanent seed implantation for localized prostate cancer. *Radiotherapy and Oncology*, 57:315–321, 2000.

7. E. Balas and M. J. Saltzman. An algorithm for the three-index assignment problem. *Operations Research*, 39:150–161, 1991.

8. L. Beaulieu, J. Pouliot, D. Tubic, and A. Zaccarin. Automated seed detection and three-dimensional reconstruction. II. Reconstruction of permanent prostate implants using simulated annealing. *Medical Physics*, 28:2272–2279, 2001.

9. P. J. Biggs and D. M. Kelley. Geometric reconstruction of seed implants using a three-film technique. *Medical Physics*, 10:701–705, 1983.

10. W. L. Brogan. Algorithm for ranked assignments with applications to multiobject tracking. *IEEE Journal of Guidance*, 12:357–364, 1989.

11. H. Chernoff. A measure of asymptotic efficiency for test of a hypothesis based on the sum of observation. *Annals of Mathematical Statistics*, 23:493–509, 1952.

12. L. M. Chin and R. L. Siddon. Two-film brachytherapy reconstruction algorithm. *Medical Physics*, 12:77–83, 1985.

13. P. S. Cho, S. T. Lam, R. J. Marks II, and S. Narayanan. 3D seed reconstruction for prostate brachytherapy using hough trajectories. *Physics in Medicine and Biology*, 49:557–569, 2004.

14. P. S. Cho, R. J. Marks, and S. Narayanan. Three-dimensional seed reconstruction from an incomplete data set for prostate brachytherapy. *Physics in Medicine and Biology*, 49:3483–3494, 2004.

15. H. Fohlin. Randomized hypergraph matching algorithms for seed reconstruction in prostate cancer radiation. Master's thesis, CAU Kiel and Göteborg University, 2005.

16. M. R. Garey and D. S. Johnson. *Computers and Intractability*. W.H. Freeman and Company, New York, 1979.

17. M. Habib, C. McDiarmid, J. Ramirez-Alfonsin, and B. Reed. *Probabilistic methods for algorithmic discrete mathematics*, volume 16 of *Springer Series in Algorithms and Combinatorics*. Springer-Verlag, 1998.

18. W. Hoeffding. Probability inequalities for sums of bounded random variables. *American Statistical Association Journal*, 58:13–30, 1963.

19. S. Janson, T. Łuczak, and A. Ruciński. *Random Graphs*. Wiley-Interscience Series in Discrete Mathematics and Optimization. John Wiley & Sons, Inc., New York, Toronto, 2000.

20. E. K. Lee, R. J. Gallagher, D. Silvern, C. S. Wu, and M. Zaider. Treatment planning for brachytherapy: an integer programming model, two computational approaches and experiments with permanent prostate implant planning. *Physics in Medicine and Biology*, 44:145–165, 1999.

21. R. Lougee-Heimer. The common optimization interface for operations research. *IBM Journal of Research and Development*, 47:75–66, 2003.

22. R. Nath and M. S. Rosenthal. An automatic seed identification technique for interstitial implants using three isocentric radiographs. *Medical Physics*, 10:475–479, 1983.

23. M. Okamoto. Some inequalities relating to the partial sum of binomial probabilities. *Annals of the Institute of Statistical Mathematics*, 10:29–35, 1958.

24. P. Raghavan and C. D. Thompson. Randomized rounding: a technique for provably good algorithms and algorithmic proofs. *Combinatorica*, 7:365–374, 1987.

25. F.-A. Siebert, P. Kohr, and G. Kovács. The design and testing of a solid phantom for the verification of a commercial 3D seed reconstruction algorithm. *Radiotherapy and Oncology*, 74:169–175, 2005.

26. F.-A. Siebert, A. Srivastav, L. Kliemann, H. Fohlin, and G. Kovács. Three-dimensional reconstruction of seed implants by randomized rounding and visual evaluation. *Medical Physics*, 34:967–957, 2007.

27. A. Srivastav. Derandomization in combinatorial optimization. In S. Rajasekaran, P. M. Pardalos, J. H. Reif, and J. D. Rolim, editors, *Handbook of Randomized Computing*, volume II, pages 731–842. Kluwer Academic Publishers, 2001.

28. A. Srivastav and P. Stangier. Algorithmic Chernoff-Hoeffding inequalities in integer programming. *Random Structures & Algorithms*, 8:27–58, 1996.

Global optimization and spatial synchronization changes prior to epileptic seizures

Shivkumar Sabesan[1], Levi Good[2], Niranjan Chakravarthy[1],
Kostas Tsakalis[1], Panos M. Pardalos[3], and Leon Iasemidis[2]

[1] Department of Electrical Engineering, Fulton School of Engineering, Arizona
State University, Tempe, AZ, 85281 shivkumar.sabesan@asu.edu,
niranjan.chakravarthy@asu.edu, tsakalis@asu.edu
[2] The Harrington Department of Bioengineering, Fulton School of Engineering,
Arizona State University, Tempe, AZ, 85281 levi.good@asu.edu,
leon.iasemidis@asu.edu.
[3] Department of Industrial and Systems Engineering, University of Florida,
Gainesville, FL, 32611 pardalos@ufl.edu

Summary. Epileptic seizures are manifestations of intermittent spatiotemporal
transitions of the human brain from chaos to order. In this paper, a comparative study involving a measure of chaos, in particular the short-term Lyapunov
exponent (STL_{max}), a measure of phase (ϕ_{max}) and a measure of energy (E) is
carried out to detect the dynamical spatial synchronization changes that precede
temporal lobe epileptic seizures. The measures are estimated from intracranial electroencephalographic (EEG) recordings with sub-dural and in-depth electrodes from
two patients with focal temporal lobe epilepsy and a total of 43 seizures. Techniques
from optimization theory, in particular quadratic bivalent programming, are applied
to optimize the performance of the three measures in detecting preictal synchronization. It is shown that spatial synchronization, as measured by the convergence
of STL_{max}, ϕ_{max} and E of critical sites selected by optimization versus randomly
selected sites leads to long-term seizure predictability. Finally, it is shown that the
seizure predictability period using STl_{max} is longer than that of the phase or energy
synchronization measures. This points out the advantages of using synchronization
of the STl_{max} measure in conjunction with optimization for long-term prediction of
epileptic seizures.

Keywords: Quadratic bivalent programming, dynamical entrainment, spatial synchronization, epileptic seizure predictability.

1 Introduction

Epilepsy is among the most common disorders of the nervous system. It occurs in all age groups, from infants to adults, and continues to be a considerable economic burden to society [6]. Temporal lobe epileptic seizures are the most common types of seizures in adults. Seizures are marked by abrupt transitions in the electroencephalographic (EEG) recordings, from irregular (chaotic) patterns before a seizure (preictal state) to more organized, rhythmic-like behavior during a seizure (ictal state), causing serious disturbances in the normal functioning of the brain [10]. The epileptiform discharges of seizures may begin locally in portions of the cerebral hemispheres (partial/focal seizures, with a single or multiple foci), or begin simultaneously in both cerebral hemispheres (primary generalized seizures). After a seizure's onset, partial seizures may remain localized and cause relatively mild cognitive, psychic, sensory, motor or autonomic symptoms (simple partial seizures), or may spread to cause altered consciousness, complex automatic behaviors, bilateral tonic-clonic (convulsive) movements (complex partial seizures) etc.. Generalized seizures cause altered consciousness at the onset and are associated with a variety of motor symptoms, ranging from brief localized body jerks to generalized tonic-clonic activity. If seizures cannot be controlled, the patient experiences major limitations in family, social, educational, and vocational activities. These limitations have profound effects on the patient's quality of life, as well as on his or her family [6]. In addition, frequent and long, uncontrollable seizures may produce irreversible damage to the brain. A condition called status epilepticus, where seizures occur continuously and the patient typically recovers only under external treatment, constitutes a life-threatening situation [9].

Until recently, the general belief in the medical community was that epileptic seizures could not be anticipated. Seizures were assumed to occur randomly over time. The 80s saw the emergence of new signal processing methodologies, based on the mathematical theory of nonlinear dynamics, optimal to deal with the spontaneous formation of organized spatial, temporal or spatiotemporal patterns in various physical, chemical and biological systems [3–5, 13, 40]. These techniques quantify the signal structure and stability from the perspective of dynamical invariants (e.g., dimensionality of the signal using the correlation dimension, or divergence of signal trajectories using the largest Lyapunov exponent), and were a drastic departure from the signal processing techniques based on the linear model (Fourier analysis). Applying these techniques on EEG data recorded from epileptic patients, a long-term, progressive, preictal dynamical change was observed [26, 27]. This observation triggered a special interest in the medical field towards early prediction of seizures with the expectation that it could lead to prevention of seizures from occurring, and therefore to a new mode of treatment for epilepsy. Medical device companies have already started off designing and implementing intervention devices for various neurodegenerative diseases (e.g., stimulators for Parkinsonian patients) in addition to the existing ones for cardiovascular applications (e.g., pacemakers, defibrillators). Along the same line, there is currently an explosion of interest for epilepsy in academic centers and medical industry, with clinical trials underway to test potential seizure prediction and intervention methodology and devices for Food and Drug Administration (FDA) approval.

In studies on seizure prediction, Iasemidis et al. [28] first reported a progressive preictal increase of spatiotemporal entrainment/synchronization among critical sites of the brain as the precursor of epileptic seizures. The algorithm used was based on the spatial convergence of short-term maximum Lyapunov exponents (STL_{max}) estimated at these critical electrode sites. Later, this observation was successfully implemented in the prospective prediction of epileptic seizures [29, 30]. The key idea in this implementation was the application of global optimization techniques for adaptive selection of groups of electrode sites that exhibit preictal (before a seizure's onset) entrainment. Seizure anticipation times of about 71.7 minutes with a false prediction rate of 0.12 per hour were reported across patients with temporal lobe epilepsy.

In the present paper, three different measures of dynamical synchronization/entrainment, namely amplitude, phase and STL_{max} are compared on the basis of their ability to detect these preictal changes. Due to the current interest in the field, and the proposed measures of energy and phase as alternatives to STL_{max} [33–36] for seizure prediction, it was deemed important to comparatively evaluate all three measures' seizure predictability (anticipation) capabilities in a retrospective study. Quadratic integer programming techniques of global optimization were applied to select critical electrode sites per measure for every recorded seizure. Results following such an analysis with 43 seizures recorded from two patients with temporal lobe epilepsy showed that: 1) Critical electrode sites selected on the basis of their synchronization per measure before a seizure outperform randomly selected ones in the ability to detect long-term preictal entrainment, and 2) critical sites selected on the basis of STL_{max} have longer and more consistent preictal trends before a majority of seizures than the ones from the other two measures of synchronization. We describe the three measures of synchronization utilized in the analysis herein in Section 2. In Section 3 we explain the formulation of a quadratic integer programming problem to select critical electrode sites for seizure prediction by each of the three measures. Statistical yardsticks used to quantify the performance of each measure in detecting preictal dynamics are given in Section 4. Results from the application of these methods to EEG are presented in Section 5, followed by conclusions in Section 6.

2 Synchronization changes prior to epileptic seizures

There has not been much of an effort to relate the measurable changes that occur before an epileptic seizure to the underlying synchronization changes that take place within areas and/or between different areas of the epileptic brain. Such information can be extracted by employing methods of spatial synchronization developed for coupled dynamical systems.

Over the past decade, different frameworks for the mathematical description of synchronization between dynamical systems have been developed, which subsequently have led to the proposition of different concepts of synchronization [12, 14, 19, 21]. Apart from the case of complete synchronization, where the state variables x_1 and x_2 of two approximately identical, strongly coupled systems 1 and 2 attain identical values ($x_1(t) = x_2(t)$), the term lag synchronization has been used to describe the case where the state variables of two interacting systems 1 and 2 attain identical values with a time lag ($x_1(t) = x_2(t + \tau)$) [42, 43]. The classical concept of phase synchronization was extended from linear to nonlinear and even chaotic systems by defining corresponding phase variables ϕ_1, ϕ_2 (see Section 2.2) [43]. The concept of generalized synchronization was introduced to cope with systems that may not be in complete, lag or phase synchronization, but nevertheless depend on each other (e.g., driver-response systems) in a more complicated manner. In this case, the state variables of the systems are connected through a particular functional relationship [2, 44]. Finally, a new type of synchronization that is more in alignment with the generalized synchronization was introduced through our work on the epileptic brain [24, 39]. We called it dynamical entrainment (or dynamical synchronization). In this type of synchronization, measures of dynamics of the systems involved attain similar values. We have shown the existence of such a behavior through measures of chaos (STL_{max}) at different locations of the epileptic brain long prior to the onset of seizures. Measures for each of these types of synchronization have been tested on models and real systems. In the following subsections, we present three of the most frequently utilized dynamical measures of EEG and compare their performance in the detection of synchronization in the epileptic human brain.

2.1 Measure of energy (E) profiles

A classical measure of a signal's strength is calculated as the sum of its amplitudes squared over a time period $T = N\Delta t$,

$$E = \sum_{k=1}^{T} x^2 (i \cdot \Delta t) \tag{1}$$

where Δt is the sampling period, $t = i \cdot \Delta t$ and x_i are the amplitude values of a scalar, real valued, sampled x signal in consideration. For EEG analysis, the Energy (E) values are calculated over consecutive non-overlapping windows of data, each window of T second in duration, from different locations in the brain over an extended period of time. Examples of E profiles over time from two electrode sites that show entrainment before a seizure are given in Figures 1(a) and 2(a) (left panels) for Patient 1 and 2 respectively. The highest

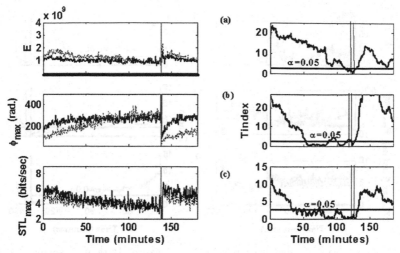

Fig. 1. Long-term synchronization prior to a seizure (Patient 1; seizure 15). **Left Panels**: (a) E profiles over time of two electrode sites (LST1, LOF2) selected to be mostly synchronized 10 min prior to the seizure. (b) ϕ_{max} profiles of two electrode sites (RST1, ROF2) selected to be mostly synchronized 10 min prior to the seizure. (c) STL_{max} profiles of two electrode sites (RTD3, LOF2) selected to be mostly synchronized 10 min prior to the seizure (seizure's onset is depicted by a vertical line). **Right Panels**: Corresponding T-index curves for the sites and measures depicted in the left panels. Vertical lines illustrate the period over which the effect of the ictal period is present in the estimation of the T-index values, since 10 min windows move forward in time every 10.24 sec over the values of the measure profiles in the left panels. Seizure lasted for 2 minutes, hence the period between vertical lines is 12 minutes.

E values were observed during the ictal period. This pattern roughly corresponds to the typical observation of higher amplitudes in the original EEG signal ictally (during a seizure). As we show below (Section 3), even though no other discernible characteristics exist in each individual E profile per electrode, synchronization trends between the E profiles across electrodes over time in the preictal period exist.

2.2 Measure of maximum phase (ϕ_{max}) profiles

The notion of phase synchronization was introduced by Huygens [22] in the 17th century for two coupled frictionless harmonic oscillators oscillating at different angular frequencies of ω_1 and ω_2 respectively, such that $\frac{\omega_1}{\omega_2} = \frac{m}{n}$. In this classical case, phase synchronization is usually defined as the locking of the phases of the two oscillators:

$$\varphi_{n,m} = n\phi_1(t) - m\phi_2(t) = constant \qquad (2)$$

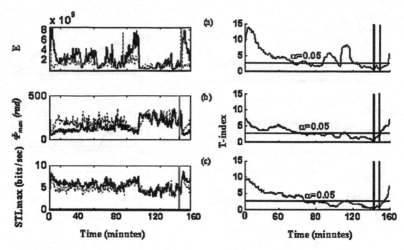

Fig. 2. Long-term synchronization prior to a seizure (Patient 2; seizure 5). **Left Panels:** (a) E profiles over time of two electrode sites (RST1, LOF2) selected to be mostly synchronized 10 min prior to the seizure. (b) ϕ_{max} profiles of two electrode sites (RTD1, LOF3) selected to be mostly synchronized 10 min prior to the seizure. (c) STL_{max} profiles of two electrode sites (RTD2, ROF3) selected to be mostly synchronized 10 min prior to the seizure (seizure's onset is depicted by a vertical line). **Right Panels:** Corresponding T-index curves for the sites and measures depicted in the left panels. Vertical lines illustrate the period over which the effect of the ictal period is present in the estimation of the T-index values, since 10 min windows move forward every 10.24 sec over the values of the measures in the left panels. Seizure lasted 3 minutes, hence the period between vertical lines is 13 minutes.

where n and m are integers, ϕ_1 and ϕ_2 denote the phases of the oscillators, and $\varphi_{n,m}$ is defined as their relative phase. In order to investigate synchronization in chaotic systems, Rosenblum et al. [42] relaxed this condition of phase locking by a weaker condition of phase synchronization (since $\frac{\omega_1}{\omega_2}$ may be an irrational real number and each system may contain power and phases at many frequencies around one dominant frequency):

$$|\varphi_{n,m}| = |n\phi_1(t) - m\phi_2(t)| < constant. \qquad (3)$$

The estimation of instantaneous phases $\phi_1(t)$ and $\phi_2(t)$ is nontrivial for many nonlinear model systems, and even more difficult when dealing with noisy time series of unknown characteristics. Different approaches have been proposed in the literature for the estimation of instantaneous phase of a signal. In the analysis that follows, we take the analytic signal approach for phase estimation [15, 38] that defines the *instantaneous phase* of an arbitrary signal $s(t)$ as

$$\phi(t) = \arctan \frac{\tilde{s}(t)}{s(t)} \qquad (4)$$

where

$$\tilde{s}(t) = \frac{1}{\pi} P.V. \int_{-\infty}^{+\infty} \frac{s(\tau)}{t-\tau} d\tau \qquad (5)$$

is the Hilbert transform of the signal $s(t)$ (P.V. denotes the Cauchy Principal Value). From Equation (5), the Hilbert transform of the signal can be interpreted as a convolution of the signal $s(t)$ with a non-causal filter $h(t) = 1/\pi t$. The Fourier transform $H(\omega)$ of $h(t)$ is $-jsgn(\omega)$ where $sgn(\omega)$ is often called the signum function and

$$sgn(\omega) = \begin{cases} 1, \, \omega > 0, \\ 0, \, \omega = 0, \\ 1, \, \omega < 0. \end{cases} \qquad (6)$$

Hence, Hilbert transformation is equivalent to a type of filtering of $s(t)$ in which amplitudes of the spectral components are left unchanged, while their phases are altered by $\pi/2$, positively or negatively according to the sign of ω. Thus, $\tilde{s}(t)$ can then be obtained by the following procedure. First, a one-sided spectrum $Z(\omega)$ in which the negative half of the spectrum is equal to zero is created by multiplying the Fourier transform $S(\omega)$ of the signal $s(t)$ with that of the filter $H(\omega)$ (i.e., $Z(\omega) = S(\omega)H(\omega)$). Next, the inverse Fourier transform of $Z(\omega)$ is computed to obtain the complex-valued "analytic" signal $z(t)$. Since $Z(\omega)$ only has a positive-sided spectrum, $z(t)$ is given by:

$$z(t) = \frac{1}{2\pi} \int_{-\infty}^{+\infty} Z(\omega)d\omega = \frac{1}{2\pi} \int_{0}^{+\infty} Z(\omega)d\omega. \qquad (7)$$

The imaginary part of $z(t)$ then yields $\tilde{s}(t)$. Mathematically, $\tilde{s}(t)$ can be compactly represented as

$$\tilde{s}(t) = -i\frac{1}{2\pi} \int_{0}^{+\infty} (S(\omega)H(\omega))d\omega. \qquad (8)$$

It is important to note that the arctangent function used to estimate the instantaneous phase in Equation (4) could be either a two-quadrant inverse tangent function (ATAN function in MATLAB) or a four-quadrant inverse tangent function (ATAN2 function in MATLAB). The ATAN function gives phase values that are restricted to the interval $[-\pi/2, +\pi/2]$ and, on exceeding the value of $+\pi/2$, fall to the value of $-\pi/2$ twice in each cycle of oscillation, while the ATAN2 function when applied to the same data gives phase values that are restricted to the interval $[-\pi, +\pi]$ and, on exceeding the value of $+\pi$, fall to the value of $-\pi$ once during every oscillation's cycle. In order to track instantaneous phase changes over long time intervals, this generated disjoint phase sequence has to be "unwrapped" [41] by adding either π, when using the ATAN function, or 2π, when using the ATAN2 function, at each phase discontinuity. Thus a continuous phase profile $\phi(t)$ over time can be generated.

The $\phi(t)$ from EEG data were estimated within non-overlapping moving windows of 10.24 seconds in duration per electrode site. Prior to the calculation of phase, to avoid edge effects in the estimation of the Fourier transform, each window was tapered with a Hamming window before Fourier transforming the data. Per window, a set of phase values are generated that are equal in number to the number of data points in this window. The maximum phase value (ϕ_{max}), minimum phase value (ϕ_{min}), mean phase value (ϕ_{mean}) and the standard deviation of the phase values (ϕ_{std}) were estimated per window. Only the dynamics of ϕ_{max} were subsequently followed over time herein, because they were found to be more sensitive than the other three phase measures to dynamical changes before seizures.

Examples of synchronized ϕ_{max} profiles over time around a seizure in Patients 1 and 2 are given in the left panels of Figures 1(b) and 2(b) respectively. The preictal, ictal and postictal states correspond to medium, high and low values of ϕ_{max} respectively. The highest ϕ_{max} values were observed during the ictal period, and higher ϕ_{max} values were observed during the preictal period than during the postictal period. This pattern roughly corresponds to the typical observation of higher frequencies in the original EEG signal ictally, and lower EEG frequencies postictally.

2.3 Measure of chaos (STL_{max}) profiles

Under certain conditions, through the method of delays described by Packard et al. [37] and Takens [46], sampling of a single variable of a system over time can determine all state variables of the system that are related to the observed state variable. In the case of the EEG, this method can be used to reconstruct a multidimensional state space of the brain's electrical activity from a single EEG channel at the corresponding brain site. Thus, in such an embedding, each state in the state space is represented by a vector $\mathbf{X}(t)$, whose components are the delayed versions of the original single-channel EEG time series $x(t)$, that is:

$$\mathbf{X}(t) = (x(t), x(t+\tau), \ldots, x(t+(d-1)\tau)) \qquad (9)$$

where τ is the time delay between successive components of $\mathbf{X}(t)$ and d is a positive integer denoting the embedding dimension of the reconstructed state space. Plotting $\mathbf{X}(t)$ in the thus created state space produces the state portrait of a spatially distributed system at the subsystem (brain's location) where $x(t)$ is recorded from. The most complicated steady state a nonlinear deterministic system can have is a strange and chaotic attractor, whose complexity is measured by its dimension D, and its chaoticity by its Kolmogorov entropy (K) and Lyapunov exponents (Ls) [16, 17]. A steady state is chaotic if at least the maximum of all Lyapunov exponents (Ls) is positive.

According to Takens, in order to properly embed a signal in the state space, the embedding dimension d should at least be equal to $(2D+1)$. Of the many different methods used to estimate D of an object in the state space, each has its own practical problems [32]. The measure most often used to estimate D is the state space correlation dimension ν. Methods for calculating ν from experimental data have been described in [1] and were employed in our work to approximate D in the ictal state. The brain, being nonstationary, is never in a steady state at any location in the strict dynamical sense. Arguably, activity at brain sites is constantly moving through "steady states," which are functions of certain parameter values at a given time. According to bifurcation theory [18], when these parameters change slowly over time, or the system is close to a bifurcation, dynamics slow down and conditions of stationarity are better satisfied. In the ictal state, temporally ordered and spatially synchronized oscillations in the EEG usually persist for a relatively long period of time (in the range of minutes). Dividing the ictal EEG into short segments ranging from 10.24 sec to 50 sec in duration, the estimation of ν from ictal EEG has produced values between 2 and 3 [25, 45], implying the existence of a low-dimensional manifold in the ictal state, which we have called "epileptic attractor." Therefore, an embedding dimension d of at least 7 has been used to properly reconstruct this epileptic attractor.

Although d of interictal (between seizures) "steady state" EEG data is expected to be higher than that of the ictal state, a constant embedding dimension $d = 7$ has been used to reconstruct all relevant state spaces over the ictal and interictal periods at different brain locations. The advantages of this approach are that a) existence of irrelevant information in dimensions higher than 7 might not influence much the estimated dynamical measures, and b) reconstruction of the state space with a low d suffers less from the short length of moving windows used to handle stationary data. The disadvantage is that relevant information to the transition to seizures in higher dimensions may not be captured.

The Lyapunov exponents measure the information flow (bits/sec) along local eigenvectors of the motion of the system within such attractors. Theoretically, if the state space is of d dimensions, we can estimate up to d Lyapunov exponents. However, as expected, only $D + 1$ of these will be real. The others are spurious [38]. Methods for calculating these dynamical measures from experimental data have been published in [26, 45]. The estimation of the largest Lyapunov exponent ($Lmax$) in a chaotic system has been shown to be more reliable and reproducible than the estimation of the remaining exponents [47], especially when D is unknown and changes over time, as in the case of high-dimensional and nonstationary EEG data. A method developed to estimate an approximation of $Lmax$ from nonstationary data is called STL (Short-term Lyapunov) [25, 26]. The STL_{max}, defined as the average of the maximum local Lyapunov exponents in the state space, can be calculated as follows:

$$STL_{max} = \frac{1}{N_a \Delta t} \sum_{i=1}^{N_a} log_2 \frac{|\delta \mathbf{X}_{i,j}(\Delta t)|}{|\delta \mathbf{X}_{i,j}(0)|} \qquad (10)$$

where $\delta\mathbf{X}_{i,j}(0) = \mathbf{X}(t_i) - \mathbf{X}(t_j)$ is the displacement vector at time t_i, that is, a perturbation of the vectors $\mathbf{X}(t_i)$ in the fiducial orbit at t_i, and $\delta\mathbf{X}_{i,j}(\Delta t) = \mathbf{X}(t_i + \Delta t) - \mathbf{X}(t_j + \Delta t)$ is the evolution of this perturbation after time Δt. Δt is the evolution time for $\delta\mathbf{X}_{i,j}$, that is, the time one allows for $\delta\mathbf{X}_{i,j}$ to evolve in the state space. Temporal and spatial constraints for the selection of the neighbor $\mathbf{X}(t_j)$ of $\mathbf{X}(t_i)$ are applied in the state space. These constraints were necessary for the algorithm to work under the presence of transients in the EEG (e.g., epileptic spikes) (for details see [25]). If the evolution time Δt is given in seconds, STL_{max} has units of bits per second. N_a is the number of local Lyapunov exponents that are estimated within a duration T of the data segment. Therefore, if Δt is the sampling period for the time domain data, $T = (N-1)\Delta t \approx N_a \Delta t - (d-1)\tau$. The STL_{max} algorithm is applied to sequential EEG epochs of 10.24 seconds recorded from electrodes in multiple brain sites to create a set of STL_{max} profiles over time (one STL_{max} profile per recording site) that characterize the spatio-temporal chaotic signature of the epileptic brain. Long-term profiles of STL_{max}, obtained by analysis of continuous EEG at two electrode sites in patients 1 and 2, are shown in the left panels of Figures 1(c) and 2(c) respectively. These figures show the evolution of STL_{max} as the brain progresses from interictal to ictal to postictal states. There is a gradual drop in STL_{max} values over tens of minutes preceding a seizure at some sites, with no observable gradual drops at other sites. The seizure is characterized by a sudden drop in STL_{max} values with a consequent steep rise in STL_{max}. This behavior of STL_{max} indicates a gradual preictal reduction in chaoticity at some sites, reaching a minimum within the seizure state, and a postictal rise in chaoticity that corresponds to the reversal of the preictal behavior. What is most interesting and consistent across seizures and patients is an observed synchronization of STL_{max} values between electrode sites prior to a seizure. We have called this phenomenon *preictal dynamical entrainment*, and it has constituted the basis for the development of epileptic seizure prediction algorithms [7, 23, 29–31].

2.4 Quantification of synchronization

A statistical distance between the values of dynamical measures at two channels i and j estimated per EEG data segment is used to quantify the synchronization between these channels. Specifically, the T_{ij} between electrode sites i and j for each measure STL_{max}, E and ϕ_{max} at time t is defined as:

$$T_{ij}^t = \frac{|\overline{D}_{ij}^t|}{\hat{\sigma}_{ij}^t/\sqrt{m}} \qquad (11)$$

where $\overline{D}_{ij}^t$ and $\hat{\sigma}_{ij}^t$ denote the sample mean and standard deviation respectively of all m differences between a measure's values at electrodes i and j within a moving window $w_t = [t - m * 10.24sec]$ over the measure profiles.

If the true mean μ_{ij}^t of the differences D_{ij}^t is equal to zero, and σ_{ij}^t are independent and normally distributed, T_{ij}^t is asymptotically distributed as the t-distribution with $(m-1)$ degrees of freedom. We have shown that these independence and normality conditions are satisfied [30]. We define desynchronization between electrode sites i and j when μ_{ij}^t is significantly different from zero at a significance level α. The desynchronization condition between the electrode sites i and j, as detected by the paired t-test, is

$$T_{ij}^t > t_{\alpha/2,m-1} = T_{th} \tag{12}$$

where $t_{\alpha/2,m-1}$ is the $100(1-\alpha/2)$ critical value of the t-distribution with $m-1$ degrees of freedom. If $T_{ij}^t \leq t_{\alpha/2,m-1}$ (which means that we do not have satisfactory statistical evidence at the α level for the differences of values of a measure between electrode sites i and j within the time window w_t to be not zero), we consider sites i and j to be synchronized with each other at time t. Using $\alpha = 0.01$ and $m = 60$, the threshold $T_{th} = 2.662$. It is noteworthy that similar STL_{max}, E or ϕ_{max} values at two electrode sites do not necessarily mean that these sites also interact. However, when there is a progressive convergence over time of the measures at these sites, the probability that they are unrelated diminishes. This is exactly what occurs before seizures, and it is illustrated in the right panels of Figures 1 and 2 for all the three measures considered herein. A progressive synchronization in all measures, as quantified by T_{ij}, is observed preictally. Note that synchronization occurs at different sites per measure. The sites per measure are selected according to the procedure described below in Section 3.

3 Optimization of spatial synchronization

Not all brain sites are progressively synchronized prior to a seizure. The selection of the ones that do (critical sites) is a global optimization problem that minimizes the distance between the dynamical measures at these sites. For many years, the Ising model [8] has been a powerful tool for studying phase transitions in statistical physics. The model is described by a graph $G(V, E)$ having n vertices $\{v_1, \ldots, v_n\}$ with each edge $e(i, j) \in E$ having a weight J_{ij} (interaction energy). Each vertex v_i has a magnetic spin variable $\sigma_i \in \{-1, +1\}$ associated with it. A spin configuration σ of minimum energy is obtained by minimizing the Hamiltonian:

$$H(\sigma) = \sum_{1 \leq i \leq j \leq n} J_{ij}\sigma_i\sigma_j \quad \text{over all } \sigma \in \{-1, +1\}^n. \tag{13}$$

This optimization problem is equivalent to the combinatorial problem of quadratic bivalent programming. Its solution gives vertices with proper spin at the global minimum energy. Motivated by the application of the Ising model to phase transitions, we have adapted quadratic bivalent (zero-one) programming techniques to optimally select the critical electrode sites during the pre-ictal transition [23, 30] that minimize the objective function of the distance of STL_{max}, E or ϕ_{max} between pairs of brain sites.

More specifically, we considered the integer bivalent 0-1 problem:

$$\min \ x^t T x \ \text{with} \ x \in (0,1)^n \quad \text{s.t.} \ \sum_{i=1}^{n} x_i = k \qquad (14)$$

where n is the total number of available electrode sites, k is the number of sites to be selected, and x_i are the (zero/one) elements of the n-dimensional vector $\mathbf{x}$. The elements of the T matrix, $T_{ij}, i = 1, \ldots, n$ and $j = 1, \ldots, n$ were previously defined in Equation (10). If the constraint in Equation (12) is included in the objective function $x^t T x$ by introducing the penalty

$$\mu = \sum_{j=1}^{n} \sum_{i=1}^{n} |T_{ij}| + 1, \qquad (15)$$

the above optimization problem in Equation (12) becomes equivalent to an unconstrained global optimization problem

$$\min \left[x^t T x + \mu \left(\sum_{i=1}^{n} x_i - k \right)^2 \right], \quad \text{where} \ x \in (0,1)^n. \qquad (16)$$

The electrode site i is selected if the corresponding element x_i^* in the n-dimensional solution x^* of Equation (14) is equal to 1.

The optimization for the selection of critical sites was performed in the preictal window $w_1(t^*) = [t^*, t^* - 10 \ min]$ over a measure's profiles, where t^* is the time of a seizure's onset, separately for each of the three considered measures. For $k = 5$, the corresponding T-index is depicted in Figures 3 and 4. After the optimal sites selection, the average T-index across all possible pairs of the selected sites is generated and followed backward in time from each seizure's onset t^*. In the following sections, for simplicity, we denote these spatially averaged T-index values by "T-index." In the estimation of the average T-index curves depicted in Figures 3 and 4 for a seizure recorded from Patients 1 and 2, the 5 critical sites selected from the E profiles were [LST1, LOF2, ROF1, RST1, ROF2] and [LST1, LOF2, LST3, RST1, RTD1]; from the STL_{max} profiles [RST1, ROF2, RTD2, RTD3, LOF2] and [RST3, LOF3, RTD3, RTD4, ROF2], and [LST2, LOF2, ROF2, RTD1, RTD2] and [LOF1, LOF2, LTD1, RST2, RTD3] from the ϕ_{max} profiles (see Figure 6 for the electrode montage). These T-index trends are then compared with the average T-index of 100 non-optimal sites, selected randomly over the space of $\binom{n}{5}$ tuples of five sites (n is the maximum amount of available recording sites). The algorithm for random selection of one tuple involves generation of $\binom{n}{5}$

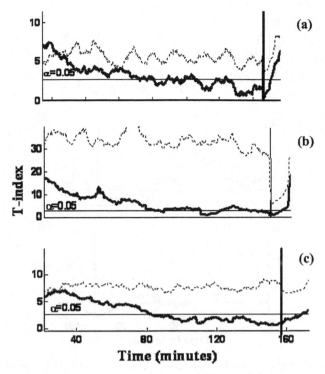

Fig. 3. Dynamical synchronization of optimal vs. non-optimal sites prior to a seizure (Patient 1; seizure 15). (a) The T-index profile generated by the E profiles of five optimal (critical) electrode sites selected by the global optimization technique 10 minutes before the seizure (solid line) and the average of the T-index profiles of 100 tuples of five randomly selected ones (non-optimal) (dotted line). (b) The T-index profile generated by the ϕ_{max} profiles of five optimal (critical) electrode sites selected by the global optimization technique 10 minutes before the seizure (solid line) and the average of the T-index profiles of 100 tuples of five randomly selected ones (non-optimal) (dotted line). (c) The T-index profile generated by the STL_{max} profiles of five optimal (critical) electrode sites selected by the global optimization technique 10 minutes before the seizure (solid line) and, for illustration purposes only, the average of the T-index profiles of 100 tuples of five randomly selected ones (non-optimal) (dotted line). Vertical lines in the figure represent the ictal state of the seizure that lasted -2 minutes.

Gaussian random numbers between 0 and 1 and reordering of the T-indices of tuples of five sites according to the order indicated by the generated random number values, and finally, selection of the top tuple from the sorted list of tuples. Repetition of the algorithm with 100 different SEEDs gives 100 different randomly selected tuples of 5 sites per seizure. For comparison purposes, the T-index profile of these non-optimal tuples of sites, averaged across all 100 randomly selected tuples of sites, is also shown in Figures 3 and 4.

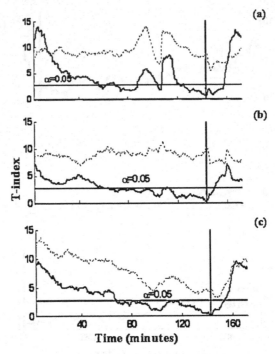

Fig. 4. Dynamical synchronization of optimal vs. non-optimal sites prior to a seizure (Patient 2; seizure 5). (a) The T-index profile generated by the E profiles of five optimal (critical) electrode sites selected by the global optimization technique 10 minutes before the seizure (solid line) and the average of the T-index profiles of 100 tuples of five randomly selected ones (non-optimal) (dotted line). (b) The T-index profile generated by the ϕ_{max} profiles of five optimal (critical) electrode sites selected by the global optimization technique 10 minutes before the seizure (solid line) and the average of the T-index profiles of 100 tuples of five randomly selected ones (non-optimal) (dotted line). (c) The T-index profile generated by the STL_{max} profiles of five optimal (critical) electrode sites selected by the global optimization technique 10 minutes before the seizure (solid line) and, for illustration purposes only, the average of the T-index profiles of 100 tuples of five randomly selected ones (non-optimal) (dotted line). Vertical lines in the figure represent the ictal state of the seizure, that lasted 3 minutes.

4 Estimation of seizure predictability time

The predictability time T_p for a given seizure is defined as the period before a seizure's onset during which synchronization between critical sites is highly statistically significant (i.e., T-index$< 2.662 = T_{th}$). Each measure of synchronization gives a different T_p for a seizure. To compensate for possible oscillations of the T-index profiles, we smooth it with a window $w_2(t)$ moving backward in time from the seizure's onset. The length of this window is the

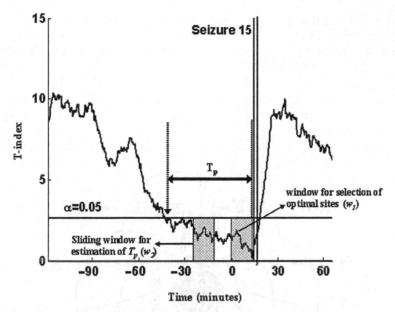

Fig. 5. Estimation of the seizure predictability time T_p. The time average T-index within the moving window $w_2(t)$ on the T-index profiles of the critical sites selected as being mostly entrained in the 10-min preictal window $w_1(t)$ is continuously estimated moving backwards from the seizure onset. When the time average T-index is $> T_{th} = 2.662$, T_p is set equal to the right endpoint of w_2.

same as the one of $w_1(t)$, in order for the T_{th} to be the same. Then T_p is estimated by the following procedure:

The time average of the T-index within a 10 minute moving window, $w_2(t) = [t, t - 10\ min]$ (the t decreases from the time t^* of the seizure's onset up to $(t^* - t) = 3\ hours$) is continuously estimated until the average of the T-index within a window $w_2(t)$ is less than or equal to T_{th}. When $t = t_0$: T-index $> T_{th}$, the $T_p = t^* - t_0$. This predictability time estimation is portrayed in Figure 5. The longer the T_p, the longer the observed synchronization prior to a seizure. Comparison of the estimated T_p by the three measures STL_{max}, E, ϕ_{max} is given in the next section.

5 Results

5.1 EEG data

A total of 43 seizures (see Table 1) from two epileptic patients with temporal lobe epilepsy were analyzed by the methodology described above. The EEG signals were recorded from six different areas of the brain by 28 electrodes (see Figure 6 for the electrode montage). Typically, 3 hours before (preictal period)

Table 1. Patients and EEG data characteristics.

Patient ID	Number of electrode sites	Location of epileptogenic focus	Seizure types	Duration of EEG recordings (days)	Number of seizures recorded
1	28	RTD	C	9.06	24
2	28	RTD	C & SC	6.07	17

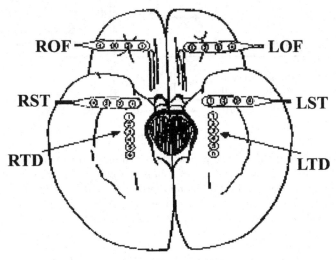

Fig. 6. Schematic diagram of the depth and subdural electrode placement. This view from the inferior aspect of the brain shows the approximate location of depth electrodes, oriented along the anterior-posterior plane in the hippocampi (RTD - right temporal depth, LTD - left temporal depth), and subdural electrodes located beneath the orbitofrontal and subtemporal cortical surfaces (ROF - right orbitofrontal, LOF left orbitofrontal, RST- right subtemporal, LST- left subtemporal).

and 1 hour after (postictal period) each seizure were analyzed with the methods described in Sections 2, 3 and 4, in search of dynamical synchronization and estimation of seizure predictability periods.

The patients in the study underwent a stereotactic placement of bilateral depth electrodes (RTD1 to RTD6 in the right hippocampus, with RTD1 adjacent to right amygdala; LTD1 to LTD6 in the left hippocampus with the LTD1 adjacent to the left amygdala; the rest of the LTD, RTD electrodes are extending posterior through the hippocampi. Two subdural strip electrodes were placed bilaterally over the orbitofrontal lobes (LOF1 to LOF4 in the left and ROF1 to ROF4 in the right lobe, with LOF1, ROF1 being most mesial and LOF4, ROF4 most lateral). Two subdural strip electrodes were placed bilaterally over the temporal lobes (LST1 to LST4 in the left and

RST1 to RST4 in the right, with LST1, RST1 being more mesial and LST4 and RST4 being more lateral). Video/EEG monitoring was performed using the Nicolet BMSI 4000 EEG machine. EEG signals were recorded using an average common reference with band pass filter settings of 0.1 Hz - 70 Hz. The data were sampled at 200Hz with a 10-bit quantization and recorded on VHS tapes continuously over days via three time-interleaved VCRs. Decoding of the data from the tapes and transfer to computer media (hard disks, DVDs, CD-ROMs) was subsequently performed off-line. The seizure predictability analysis also was performed retrospectively (off-line).

5.2 Predictability of epileptic seizures

For each of the 43 recorded seizures, the five most synchronized sites were selected within 10 minutes (window $w_1(t)$) prior to each seizure onset by the optimization procedure described in Section 3 (critical sites). The spatially averaged T-index profiles over these critical sites were estimated per seizure. Then, the predictability time of T_p for each seizure and dynamical measure, according to the procedure described in Section 4, was estimated. Using Equation (15), predictability times were obtained for all 43 recorded seizures from the two patients for each of the three dynamical measures. The algorithm for estimation of T_p delivered visually agreeable predictability times for all profiles that decrease in a near-monotonic fashion. The average predictability time obtained across seizures in our analysis for Patients 1 and 2 were 61.6 and 71.69 minutes respectively (see Table 3). The measure of classical energy, applied to single EEG channels, was shown before to lack consistent predicative ability for a seizure [11, 20]. Furthermore, its predictive performance was shown to deteriorate by postictal changes and changes during sleep-wake cycles [34]. By studying the spatiotemporal synchronization of the energy profiles between multiple EEG signals, we found average predictability times of 13.72 and 27.88 minutes for Patients 1 and 2 respectively, a significant improvement in their performance over what has been reported in the literature. For the measure of phase synchronization, the average predictability time values were 39.09 and 47.33 minutes for Patients 1 and 2 respectively. The study of the performance of all the three measures in a prospective fashion (prediction) is currently underway.

Improved predictability via global optimization

Figures 3 and 4 show the T-index profiles generated by STL_{max}, E and ϕ_{max} profiles (solid line) of five optimal (critical) electrode sites selected by the global optimization technique and five randomly selected ones (non-optimal) (dotted line) before a seizure. In these figures, a trend of T-index profiles toward low values (synchronization) can be observed preictally only when optimal sites were selected for a synchronization measure. The null hypothesis that the obtained average value of T_p from the optimal sites across all seizures is statistically smaller or equal to the average T_p from the randomly selected ones was then tested. T_p values were obtained for a total of 100 randomly selected tuples of five sites per seizure per measure. Using a two-sample t-test for every measure, the null hypothesis that the T_{popt} values (Average T_p values obtained from optimal electrode sites) were greater than the mean of the $T_{prandom}$ values (Average T_p values obtained from randomly selected electrode sites) was tested at $\alpha = 0.01$ (2422 degrees of freedom for the t-test in Patient 1, that is 100 random tuples of sites per seizure for all 24 seizures - 1 (2399 degrees of freedom) + one optimal tuple of sites per seizure for all 24 seizures-1 (23 degrees of freedom); similarly 1917 degrees of freedom for Patient 2). The T_{popt} values were significantly larger than the $T_{prandom}$ values for all three measures (see Tables 2 and 3). This result was consistent across both patients and further supports the hypothesis that the spatiotemporal dynamics of synchronization of critical (optimal) brain sites per synchronization measure should be followed in time to observe significant preictal changes predictive of an upcoming seizure.

Table 2. Mean and standard deviation of seizure predictability time T_p of 100 groups of five randomly selected sites per seizure and measure in Patients 1 and 2.

	$T_{prandom}(minutes)$			
Measure	**Patient 1**(24 seizures)		**Patient 2**(19 seizures)	
	Mean	*std.*	*Mean*	*std.*
STL_{max}	7.60	9.50	10.69	12.62
E	6.72	7.10	7.98	8.97
ϕ_{max}	7.09	6.05	7.03	9.04

Table 3. Mean and standard deviation of seizure predictability time T_p of optimal sites per measure across all seizures in Patients 1 and 2. Statistical comparison with T_p from 100 groups of non-optimal sites.

	$T_{popt}(minutes)$					
Measure	**Patient 1**(24 seizures)			**Patient 2**(19 seizures)		
	Mean	*std.*	$P\,(T_{popt} \leq T_{prandom})$	*Mean*	*std.*	$P\,(T_{popt} \leq T_{prandom})$
STL_{max}	61.60	45.50	$P < 0.0005$	71.69	33.62	$P < 0.0005$
E	13.72	11.50	$P < 0.002$	27.88	26.97	$P < 0.004$
ϕ_{max}	39.09	20.88	$P < 0.0005$	47.33	33.34	$P < 0.0005$

Comparative performance of energy, phase and STL_{max} measures in detection of preictal synchronization

Dynamical synchronization using STL_{max} consistently resulted to longer predictability times T_p than the ones by the other two measures (See Table 3). Among the other two measures, the phase synchronization measure outperformed the linear, energy-based measure and, for some seizures, it even had comparable performance to that of STL_{max}-based synchronization. These results are consistent with the synchronization observed in coupled non-identical chaotic oscillator models: an increase in coupling between two oscillators initiates generalized synchronization (best detected by STL_{max}), followed by phase synchronization (detected by phase measures), and upon further increase in coupling, amplitude synchronization (detected by energy measures) [2, 14, 42, 43].

6 Conclusion

The results of this study show that the analyzed epileptic seizures could be predicted only if optimization and synchronization were combined. The key underlying principle for such a methodology is the existence of dynamical entrainment among critical sites of the epileptic brain prior to seizures. Synchronization of non-critical sites does not show any statistical significance for seizure prediction and inclusion of these sites may mask the phenomenon. This study suggests that it may be possible to predict focal-onset epileptic seizures by analysis of linear, as well as nonlinear, measures of dynamics of multichannel EEG signals (namely the energy, phase and Lyapunov exponents), but at different time scales.

Previous studies by our group have shown that a preictal transition exists, in which the values of the maximum Lyapunov exponents (STL_{max}) of EEG recorded from critical electrode sites converge long before a seizure's onset [26]. The electrode sites involved in such a dynamical spatiotemporal interaction vary from seizure to seizure even in the same patient. Thus, the ability to predict a given seizure depends upon the ability to identify the critical electrode sites that participate in the preictal period of that seizure. Similar conclusions can be derived from the spatiotemporal analysis of the EEG with the measures of energy and phase employed herein.

By applying a quadratic zero-one optimization technique for the selection of critical brain sites from the estimated energy and the maximum phase profiles, we demonstrated that mean predictability times of 13 to 20 minutes for the energy and 36 to 43 minutes for the phase are attained, which are smaller than the ones obtained from the employment of the STL_{max} measure. For example, the mean predictability time across the two patients for the measure of phase (43.21 minutes) and energy (20.88 minutes) was worse than that of the STLmax (66.64 minutes). In the future, we plan to further study the observed spatiotemporal synchronization and the long-term predictability periods before seizures. For example, it would be worthy to investigate if similar synchronization exists at time points of the EEG recordings unrelated to the progression to seizures. Such a study will address how specific our present findings are to epileptic seizures. The proposed measures may also become valuable for on-line, real-time seizure prediction. Such techniques could be incorporated into diagnostic and therapeutic devices for long-term monitoring and treatment of epilepsy. Potential diagnostic applications include a seizure warning system from long-term EEG recordings in a hospital setting (e.g., in a diagnostic epilepsy monitoring unit). This type of system could be used to timely warn the patient or professional staff of an impending seizure in order to take precaution measures or to trigger certain preventive action. Also, such a seizure warning algorithm, being implemented in digital signal processing chips, could be incorporated into implantable therapeutic devices to timely activate deep brain stimulators (DBS) or implanted drug-release reservoirs to interrupt the route of the epileptic brain towards seizures. These types of devices, if they are adequately sensitive and specific to impending seizures, could revolutionize the treatment of epilepsy.

Acknowledgement

This project was supported by the Epilepsy Research Foundation and the Ali Paris Fund for LKS Research and Education, and National Institutes of Health (R01EB002089).

References

1. H. D. I. Abarbanel. *Analysis of Observed Chaotic Data*. Springer Verlag, 1996.
2. V. S. Afraimovich, N. N. Verichev, and M. I. Rabinovich. General synchronization. *Radiophysics and Quantum Electronics*, 29:747, 1986.
3. A. M. Albano, A. I. Mees, G. C. de Guzman, P. E. Rapp, H. Degn, A. Holden, and L. F. Isen. Chaos in biological systems, 1987.
4. A. Babloyantz and A. Destexhe. Low-Dimensional Chaos in an Instance of Epilepsy. *Proceedings of the National Academy of Sciences*, 83:3513–3517, 1986.
5. H. Bai-Lin. *Directions in Chaos Vol. 1*. World Scientific Press, 1987.
6. C. E. Begley and E. Beghi. Laboratory Research The Economic Cost of Epilepsy: A Review of the Literature. *Epilepsia*, 43:3–10, 2002.
7. W. Chaovalitwongse, L. D. Iasemidis, P. M. Pardalos, P. R. Carney, D. S. Shiau, and J. C. Sackellares. Performance of a seizure warning algorithm based on the dynamics of intracranial EEG. *Epilepsy Research*, 64:93–113, 2005.
8. C. Domb and M. S. Green. *Phase Transitions and Critical Phenomena*. Academic Press, New York, 1974.
9. J. Engel. *Seizures and Epilepsy*. FA Davis, 1989.

10. J. Engel Jr, P. D. Williamson, and H. G. Wieser. Mesial temporal lobe epilepsy. *Epilepsy: a comprehensive textbook. Philadelphia: Lippincott-Raven*, pages 2417–2426, 1997.

11. R. Esteller, J. Echauz, M. D'Alessandro, G. Worrell, S. Cranstoun, G. Vachtsevanos, and B. Litt. Continuous energy variation during the seizure cycle: towards an on-line accumulated energy. *Clin Neurophysiol*, 116:517–26, 2005.

12. L. Fabiny, P. Colet, R. Roy, and D. Lenstra. Coherence and phase dynamics of spatially coupled solid-state lasers. *Physical Review A*, 47:4287–4296, 1993.

13. W. J. Freeman. Simulation of chaotic EEG patterns with a dynamic model of the olfactory system. *Biological Cybernetics*, 56:139–150, 1987.

14. H. Fujisaka and T. Yamada. Stability theory of synchronized motion in coupled-oscillator systems. *Prog. Theor. Phys*, 69:32–47, 1983.

15. D. Gabor. Theory of communication. *Proc. IEE London*, 93:429–457, 1946.

16. P. Grassberger and I. Procaccia. Characterization of Strange Attractors. *Physical Review Letters*, 50:346–349, 1983.

17. P. Grassberger and I. Procaccia. Measuring the strangeness of strange attractors. *Physica D: Nonlinear Phenomena*, 9:189–208, 1983.

18. H. Haken. *Principles of Brain Functioning: A Synergetic Approach to Brain Activity, Behavior and Cognition.* Springer–Verlag, Berlin, 1996.

19. S. K. Han, C. Kurrer, and Y. Kuramoto. Dephasing and Bursting in Coupled Neural Oscillators. *Physical Review Letters*, 75:3190–3193, 1995.

20. M. A. Harrison, M. G. Frei, and I. Osorio. Accumulated energy revisited. *Clin Neurophysiol*, 116(3):527–31, 2005.

21. J. F. Heagy, T. L. Carroll, and L. M. Pecora. Synchronous chaos in coupled oscillator systems. *Physical Review E*, 50:1874–1885, 1994.

22. C. Hugenii. Horoloquim Oscilatorium. *Paris: Muguet. Reprinted in English as: The pendulum clock. Ames, IA: Iowa State UP*, 1986.

23. L. D. Iasemidis, P. Pardalos, J. C. Sackellares, and D. S. Shiau. Quadratic Binary Programming and Dynamical System Approach to Determine the Predictability of Epileptic Seizures. *Journal of Combinatorial Optimization*, 5:9–26, 2001.

24. L. D. Iasemidis, A. Prasad, J. C. Sackellares, P. M. Pardalos, and D. S. Shiau. On the prediction of seizures, hysteresis and resetting of the epileptic brain: insights from models of coupled chaotic oscillators. *Order and Chaos, T. Bountis and S. Pneumatikos, Eds. Thessaloniki, Greece: Publishing House K. Sfakianakis*, 8:283–305, 2003.

25. L. D. Iasemidis, J. C. Principe, and J. C. Sackellares. Measurement and quantification of spatio-temporal dynamics of human epileptic seizures. In M. Akay, editor, *Nonlinear Biomedical Signal Processing*, volume II, pages 294–318. IEEE Press, 2000.

26. L. D. Iasemidis and J. C. Sackellares. The temporal evolution of the largest Lyapunov exponent on the human epileptic cortex. *Measuring Chaos in the Human Brain. Singapore: World Scientific*, pages 49–82, 1991.

27. L. D. Iasemidis and J. C. Sackellares. Chaos theory and epilepsy. *The Neuroscientist*, 2:118–125, 1996.

28. L. D. Iasemidis, J. C. Sackellares, H. P. Zaveri, and W. J. Williams. Phase space topography of the electrocorticogram and the Lyapunov exponent in partial seizures. *Brain Topography*, 2:187–201, 1990.

29. L. D. Iasemidis, D. S. Shiau, W. Chaovalitwongse, P. M. Pardalos, P. R. Carney, and J. C. Sackellares. Adaptive seizure prediction system. *Epilepsia*, 43:264–265, 2002.

30. L. D. Iasemidis, D. S. Shiau, W. Chaovalitwongse, J. C. Sackellares, P. M. Pardalos, J. C. Principe, P. R. Carney, A. Prasad, B. Veeramani, and K. Tsakalis. Adaptive epileptic seizure prediction system. *IEEE Transactions on Biomedical Engineering*, 50:616–627, 2003.

31. L. D. Iasemidis, D. S. Shiau, P. M. Pardalos, W. Chaovalitwongse, K. Narayanan, A. Prasad, K. Tsakalis, P. R. Carney, and J. C. Sackellares. Long-term prospective on-line real-time seizure prediction. *Clin Neurophysiol*, 116:532–44, 2005.

32. Eric J. Kostelich. Problems in estimating dynamics from data. *Physica D: Nonlinear Phenomena*, 58:138–152, 1992.

33. M. Le Van Quyen, J. Martinerie, V. Navarro, P. Boon, M. D'Havé, C. Adam, B. Renault, F. Varela, and M. Baulac. Anticipation of epileptic seizures from standard EEG recordings. *The Lancet*, 357:183–188, 2001.

34. B. Litt, R. Esteller, J. Echauz, M. D'Alessandro, R. Shor, T. Henry, P. Pennell, C. Epstein, R. Bakay, M. Dichter, et al. Epileptic Seizures May Begin Hours in Advance of Clinical Onset A Report of Five Patients. *Neuron*, 30:51–64, 2001.

35. F. Mormann, T. Kreuz, R. G. Andrzejak, P. David, K. Lehnertz, and C. E. Elger. Epileptic seizures are preceded by a decrease in synchronization. *Epilepsy Research*, 53:173–185, 2003.

36. I. Osorio, M. G. Frei, and S. B. Wilkinson. Real-time automated detection and quantitative analysis of seizures and short-term prediction of clinical onset. *Epilepsia*, 39:615–627, 1998.

37. N. H. Packard, J. P. Crutchfield, J. D. Farmer, and R. S. Shaw. Geometry from a Time Series. *Physical Review Letters*, 45:712–716, 1980.

38. P.F. Panter. *Modulation, noise, and spectral analysis: applied to information transmission.* McGraw-Hill, 1965.

39. A. Prasad, L. D. Iasemidis, S. Sabesan, and K. Tsakalis. Dynamical hysteresis and spatial synchronization in coupled non-identical chaotic oscillators. *Pramana–Journal of Physics*, 64:513–523, 2005.

40. L. Rensing, U. an der Heiden, and M. C. Mackey. *Temporal Disorder in Human Oscillatory Systems: Proceedings of an International Symposium, University of Bremen, 8-13 September 1986.* Springer-Verlag, 1987.

41. M. G. Rosenblum and J. Kurths. Analysing synchronization phenomena from bivariate data by means of the Hilbert transform. In H. Kantz, J. Kurths, and G. Mayer-Kress, editors, *Nonlinear Analysis of Physiological Data*, pages 91–99. Springer, Berlin, 1998.

42. M. G. Rosenblum, A. S. Pikovsky, and J. Kurths. Phase Synchronization of Chaotic Oscillators. *Physical Review Letters*, 76:1804–1807, 1996.

43. M. G. Rosenblum, A. S. Pikovsky, and J. Kurths. From Phase to Lag Synchronization in Coupled Chaotic Oscillators. *Physical Review Letters*, 78:4193–4196, 1997.

44. N. F. Rulkov, M. M. Sushchik, L. S. Tsimring, and H. D. I. Abarbanel. Generalized synchronization of chaos in directionally coupled chaotic systems. *Physical Review E*, 51:980–994, 1995.

45. J. C. Sackellares, L. D. Iasemidis, D. S. Shiau, R. L. Gilmore, and S. N. Roper. Epilepsy when chaos fails. *Chaos in the brain?* K. Lehnertz, J. Arnhold,

P. Grassberger and C. E. Elger, Eds. Singapore: World Scientific, pages 112–133, 2000.

46. F. Takens. Detecting strange attractors in turbulence. In D. A. Rand and L. S. Young, editors, *Dynamical Systems and Turbulence, Lecture Notes in Mathematics.* Springer–Verlag, Heidelburg, 1991.

47. J. A. Vastano and E. J. Kostelich. Comparison of algorithms for determining lyapunov exponents from experimental data. In G. Mayer-Press, editor, *Dimensions and entropies in chaotic systems: quantification of complex behavior.* Springer–Verlag, 1986.

Optimization-based predictive models in medicine and biology

Eva K. Lee[1,2,3]

[1] Center for Operations Research in Medicine and HealthCare, School of Industrial and Systems Engineering, Georgia Institute of Technology, Atlanta, Georgia 30332-0205 eva.lee@isye.gatech.edu
[2] Center for Bioinformatics and Computational Genomics, Georgia Institute of Technology, Atlanta, Georgia 30332
[3] Winship Cancer Institute, Emory University School of Medicine, Atlanta, GA 30322

Summary. We present novel optimization-based classification models that are general purpose and suitable for developing predictive rules for large heterogeneous biological and medical data sets. Our predictive model simultaneously incorporates (1) the ability to classify any number of distinct groups; (2) the ability to incorporate heterogeneous types of attributes as input; (3) a high-dimensional data transformation that eliminates noise and errors in biological data; (4) the ability to incorporate constraints to limit the rate of misclassification, and a reserved-judgment region that provides a safeguard against over-training (which tends to lead to high misclassification rates from the resulting predictive rule); and (5) successive multi-stage classification capability to handle data points placed in the reserved judgment region. Application of the predictive model to a broad class of biological and medical problems is described. Applications include: the differential diagnosis of the type of erythemato-squamous diseases; genomic analysis and prediction of aberrant CpG island meythlation in human cancer; discriminant analysis of motility and morphology data in human lung carcinoma; prediction of ultrasonic cell disruption for drug delivery; identification of tumor shape and volume in treatment of sarcoma; multistage discriminant analysis of biomarkers for prediction of early atherosclerosis; fingerprinting of native and angiogenic microvascular networks for early diagnosis of diabetes, aging, macular degeneracy and tumor metastasis, and prediction of protein localization sites. In all these applications, the predictive model yields correct classification rates ranging from 80% to 100%. This provides motivation for pursuing its use as a medical diagnostic, monitoring and decision-making tool.

Keywords: Classification, prediction, predictive health, discriminant analysis, machine learning, discrete support vector machine, multi-category classification models, optimization, integer programming, medical diagnosis.

1 Introduction

A fundamental problem in discriminant analysis, or supervised learning, concerns the classification of an entity into one of $G(G \geq 2)$ a priori, mutually exclusive groups based upon k specific measurable features of the entity. Typically, a discriminant rule is formed from data collected on a sample of entities for which the group classifications are known. Then new entities, whose classifications are unknown, can be classified based on this rule. Such an approach has been applied in a variety of domains, and a large body of literature on both the theory and applications of discriminant analysis exists (e.g., see the bibliography in [60]).

In experimental biological and medical research, very often, experiments are performed and measurements are recorded under different conditions and/or on different cells/molecules. A critical analysis involves the discrimination of different features under different conditions that will reveal potential predictors for biological and medical phenomena. Hence, classification techniques play an extremely important role in biological analysis, as they facilitate systematic correlation and classification of different biological and medical phenomena. A resulting predictive rule can assist, for example, in early disease prediction and diagnosis, identification of new target sites (genomic, cellular, molecular) for treatment and drug delivery, disease prevention and early intervention, and optimal treatment design.

There are five fundamental steps in discriminant analysis: a) Determine the data for input and the predictive output classes. b) Gather a training set of data (including output class) from human experts or from laboratory experiments. Each element in the training set is an entity with a corresponding known output class. c) Determine the input attributes to represent each entity. d) Identify discriminatory attributes and develop the predictive rule(s); e) Validate the performance of the predictive rule(s).

In our Center for Operations Research in Medicine, we have developed a general-purpose discriminant analysis modeling framework and computational engine for various biological and biomedical informatics analyses. Our model, the first discrete support vector machine, offers distinct features (e.g., the ability to classify any number of groups, management of the curse of dimensionality in data attributes, and a reserved judgment region to facilitate multi-stage classification analysis) that are not simultaneously available in existing classification software [27, 28, 49, 42, 43]. Studies involving tumor volume identification, ultrasonic cell disruption in drug delivery, lung tumor cell motility analysis, CpG island aberrant methylation in human cancer, predicting early atherosclerosis using biomarkers, and fingerprinting native and angiogenic microvascular networks using functional perfusion data indicate that our approach is adaptable and can produce effective and reliable predictive rules for various biomedical and bio-behavior phenomena [14, 22, 23, 44, 46, 48, 50].

Section 2 briefly describes the background of discriminant analysis. Section 3 describes the optimization-based multi-stage discriminant analysis predictive models for classification. The use of the predictive models on various biological and medical problems are presented in Section 4. This is followed by a brief summary in Section 5.

2 Background

The main objective in discriminant analysis is to derive rules that can be used to classify entities into groups. Discriminant rules are typically expressed in terms of variables representing a set of measurable attributes of the entities in question. Data on a sample of entities for which the group classifications are known (perhaps determined by extraordinary means) are collected and used to derive rules that can be used to classify new yet-to-be-classified entities. Often there is a trade-off between the discriminating ability of the selected attributes and the expense of obtaining measurements on these attributes. Indeed, the measurement of a relatively definitive discriminating feature may be prohibitively expensive to obtain on a routine basis, or perhaps impossible to obtain at the time that classification is needed.

Thus, a discriminant rule based on a selected set of feature attributes will typically be an imperfect discriminator, sometimes misclassifying entities. Depending on the application, the consequences of misclassifying an entity may be substantial. In such a case, it may be desirable to form a discrimination rule that allows less specific classification decisions, or even non-classification of some entities, to reduce the probability of misclassification.

To address this concern, a number of researchers have suggested methods for deriving *partial discrimination rules* [10, 31, 35, 63, 65]. A partial discrimination rule allows an entity to be classified into some subset of the groups (i.e., rule out membership in the remaining groups), or be placed in a "reserved-judgement" category. An entity is considered misclassified only when it is assigned to a nonempty subset of groups not containing the true group of the entity. Typically, methods for deriving partial discrimination rules attempt to constrain the misclassification probabilities (e.g., by enforcing an upper bound on the proportion of misclassified training sample entities). For this reason, the resulting rules are also sometimes called *constrained discrimination rules*.

Partial (or constrained) discrimination rules are intuitively appealing. A partial discrimination rule based on relatively inexpensive measurements can be tried first. If the rule classifies the entity satisfactorily according to the needs of the application, then nothing further needs to be done. Otherwise, additional measurements — albeit more expensive — can be taken on other, more definitive, discriminating attributes of the entity.

One disadvantage of partial discrimination methods is that there is no obvious definition of optimality among any set of rules satisfying the constraints on the misclassification probabilities. For example, since some correct classifications are certainly more valuable than others (e.g., classification into a small subset containing the true group versus a large subset), it does not make sense to simply maximize the probability of correct classification. In fact, to maximize the probability of correct classification, one would merely classify every entity into the subset consisting of all the groups — clearly, not an acceptable rule.

A simplified model, whereby one incorporates only the reserved-judgment region (i.e., an entity is either classified as belonging to exactly one of the given a priori groups, or it is placed in the reserved-judgment category), is amenable to reasonable notions of optimality. For example, in this case, maximizing the probability of correct classification is meaningful. For the two-group case, the simplified model and the more general model are equivalent. Research on the two-group case is summarized in [60]. For three or more groups, the two models are not equivalent, and most work has been directed towards the development of heuristic methods for the more general model (e.g., see [10, 31, 63, 65]).

Assuming that the group density functions and prior probabilities are known, the author in [1] showed that an optimal rule for the problem of maximizing the probability of correct classification subject to constraints on the misclassification probabilities must be of a specific form when discriminating among multiple groups with a simplified model. The formulae in Anderson's result depend on a set of parameters satisfying a complex relationship between the density functions, the prior probabilities, and the bounds on the misclassification probabilities. Establishing a viable mathematical model to describe Anderson's result, and finding values for these parameters that yield an optimal rule are challenging tasks. The authors in [27, 28] presented the first computational model for Anderson's results.

A variety of mathematical-programming models have been proposed for the discriminant-analysis problem [2–4, 15, 24, 25, 30, 32–34, 37, 54, 56, 58, 64, 70, 71]. None of these studies deal formally with measuring the performance of discriminant rules specifically designed to allow allocation to a reserved-judgment region. There is also no mechanism employed to constrain the level of misclassifications for each group.

Many different techniques and methodologies have contributed to advances in classification, including artificial neural networks, decision trees, kernel-based learning, machine learning, mathematical programming, statistical analysis, and support vector machines [5, 8, 19, 20, 55, 61, 73]. There are some review papers for classification problems with mathematical programming techniques. The author in [69] summarizes basic concepts and ideas and discusses potential research directions on classification methods that optimize a function of the L_p-norm distances. The paper focuses on continuous models and includes normalization schemes, computational aspects, weighted formulations, secondary criteria, and extensions from two-group to multigroup classifications. The authors in [77] review the research conducted on the framework of the multicriteria decision aiding, covering different classification models. The author in [57] and the authors in [7] give an overview of using mathematical programming approaches to solve data mining problems. Most recently, the authors in [53] provide a comprehensive overview of continuous and discrete mathematical programming models for classification problems.

3 Discrete support vector machine predictive models

Since 1997, we have been developing in our computational center a general-purpose discriminant analysis modeling framework and a computational engine that is applicable to a wide variety of applications, including biological, biomedical and logistics problems. Utilizing the technology of large-scale discrete optimization and support-vector machines, we have developed novel predictive models that simultaneously include the following features: 1) the ability to classify any number of distinct groups; 2) the ability to incorporate heterogeneous types of attributes as input; 3) a high-dimensional data transformation that eliminates noise and errors in biological data; 4) constraints to limit the rate of misclassification, and a reserved-judgment region that provides a safeguard against over-training (which tends to lead to high misclassification rates from the resulting predictive rule); and 5) successive multi-stage classification capability to handle data points placed in the reserved judgment region. Based on the descriptions in [27, 28, 42, 43, 49], we summarize below some of the classification models we have developed.

3.1 Modeling of reserved-judgment region for general groups

When the population densities and prior probabilities are known, the constrained rules with a reject option (reserved-judgment), based on Anderson's results, calls for finding a partition $\{R_0, ..., R_G\}$ of $\mathbb{R}^k$ that maximizes the probability of correct allocation subject to constraints on the misclassification probabilities; i.e.,

$$\max \quad \sum_{g=1}^{G} \pi_g \int_{R_g} f_g(w)\, dw \tag{1}$$

$$\text{s.t.} \quad \int_{R_g} f_h(w) dw \leq \alpha_{hg}, \; h, \; g = 1, ..., G, \; h \neq g, \tag{2}$$

where f_h, $h = 1, ..., G$, are the group conditional density functions, π_g denotes the prior probability that a randomly selected entity is from group g, $g = 1, ..., G$, and α_{hg}, $h \neq g$ are constants between zero and one. Under quite general assumptions, it was shown that there exist unique (up to a set of measure zero) nonnegative constants λ_{ih}, $i, h \in \{1, ..., G\}$, $i \neq h$, such that the optimal rule is given by

$$R_g = \{x \in \mathbb{R}^k : L_g(x) = \max_{h \in \{0,1,...,G\}} L_h(x)\}, \; g = 0, ..., G \tag{3}$$

where

$$L_0(x) = 0 \qquad (4)$$

$$L_h(x) = \pi_h f_h(x) - \sum_{i=1, i \neq h}^{G} \lambda_{ih} f_i(x), \quad h = 1, ..., G. \qquad (5)$$

For $G = 2$ the optimal solution can be modeled in a rather straightforward manner. However, finding optimal λ_{ih}'s for the general case $G \geq 3$ is a difficult problem, with the difficulty increasing as G increases. Our model offers an avenue for modeling and finding the optimal solution in the general case. It is the first such model to be computationally viable [27, 28].

Before proceeding, we note that R_g can be written as $R_g = \{x \in \mathbb{R}^k : L_g(x) \geq L_h(x)$ for all $h = 0, ..., G\}$. So, since $L_g(x) \geq L_h(x)$ if, and only if, $(1/\sum_{t=1}^{G} f_t(x))L_g(x) \geq (1/\sum_{t=1}^{G} f_t(x))L_h(x)$, the functions L_h, $h = 1, ..., G$ can be redefined as

$$L_h(x) = \pi_h p_h(x) - \sum_{i=1, i \neq h}^{G} \lambda_{ih} p_i(x), \quad h = 1, ..., G \qquad (6)$$

where $p_i(x) = f_i(x) / \sum_{t=1}^{G} f_t(x)$. We assume that L_h is defined as in equation (6) in our model.

3.2 Mixed integer programming formulations

Assume that we are given a training sample of N entities whose group classifications are known; say n_g entities are in group g, where $\sum_{g=1}^{G} n_g = N$. Let the k dimensional vectors x^{gj}, $g = 1, ..., G$, $j = 1, ..., n_g$, contain the measurements on k available characteristics of the entities. Our procedure for deriving a discriminant rule proceeds in two stages. The first stage is to use the training sample to compute estimates, $\hat{f}_h$, either parametrically or non-parametrically, of the density functions f_h (e.g., see [60]) and estimates, $\hat{\pi}_h$, of the prior probabilities π_h, $h = 1, ..., G$. The second stage is to determine the optimal λ_{ih}s given these estimates. This stage requires being able to estimate the probabilities of correct classification and misclassification for any candidate set of λ_{ih}s. One could, in theory, substitute the estimated densities and prior probabilities into equations (5), and directly use the resulting regions R_g in the integral expressions given in (1) and (2). This would involve, even in simple cases such as normally distributed groups, the numerical evaluation of k-dimensional integrals at each step of a search for the optimal λ_{ih}s. Therefore, we have designed an alternative approach. After substituting the $\hat{f}_h$s and $\hat{\pi}_h$s into equation (5), we simply calculate the proportion of training sample points which fall in each of the regions $R_1, ..., R_G$. The mixed integer programming (MIP) models discussed below attempt to maximize the proportion of training sample points correctly classified while satisfying constraints on the proportions of training sample points misclassified. This approach has two advantages. First, it avoids having to evaluate the potentially difficult integrals in Equations (1) and (2). Second, it is nonparametric in controlling the training sample misclassification probabilities. That is, even if the densities are poorly estimated (by assuming, for example, normal densities for non-normal data), the constraints are still satisfied for the training sample. Better estimates of the densities may allow a higher correct classification rate to be achieved, but the constraints will be satisfied even if poor estimates are used. Unlike most support vector machine models that minimize the sum of errors, our objective is driven by the number of correct classifications, and will not be biased by the distance of the entities from the supporting hyperplane.

A word of caution is in order. In traditional unconstrained discriminant analysis, the true probability of correct classification of a given discriminant rule tends to be smaller than the rate of correct classification for the training sample from which it was derived. One would expect to observe such an effect for the method described herein as well as an analogous effect with regard to constraints on misclassification probabilities — the true probabilities are likely to be greater than any limits imposed on the proportions of training sample misclassifications. Hence, the α_{hg} parameters should be carefully chosen for the application in hand.

Our first model is a nonlinear 0/1 MIP model with the nonlinearity appearing in the constraints. Model 1 maximizes the number of correct classifications of the given N training entities. Similarly, the constraints on the misclassification probabilities are modeled by ensuring that the number of group g training entities in region R_h is less than or equal to a pre-specified percentage, $\alpha_{hg}(0 < \alpha_{hg} < 1)$, of the total number, n_g, of group g entities, $h, g \in \{1, ..., G\}$, $h \neq g$.

For notational convenience, let $\mathbf{G} = \{1, ..., G\}$ and $\mathbf{N}_g = \{1, ..., n_g\}$, for $g \in \mathbf{G}$. Also, analogous to the definition of p_i, define $\hat{p}_i$ by $\hat{p}_i = \hat{f}_i(x) / \sum_{t=1}^{G} \hat{f}_t(x)$. In our model, we use binary indicator variables to denote the group classification of entities. Mathematically, let u_{hgj} be a binary variable indicating whether or not x^{gj} lies in region R_h; i.e., whether or not the jth entity from group g is allocated to group h. Then Model 1 can be written as follows:

$$\max \quad \sum_{g \in G} \sum_{j \in N_g} u_{ggj}$$

s.t.

$$L_{hgj} = \hat{\pi}_h \hat{p}_h(x^{gj}) - \sum_{i \in G \setminus h} \lambda_{ih} \hat{p}_i(x^{gj}), \quad h, g \in \mathbf{G}, \ j \in \mathbf{N}_g \qquad (7)$$

$$y_{gj} = \max\{0, L_{hgj} : h = 1, ..., G\}, \qquad g \in \mathbf{G}, \ j \in \mathbf{N}_g \qquad (8)$$

$$y_{gj} - L_{ggj} \leq M(1 - u_{ggj}), \qquad g \in \mathbf{G}, \ j \in \mathbf{N}_g \qquad (9)$$

$$y_{gj} - L_{hgj} \geq \varepsilon(1 - u_{hgj}), \qquad h, g \in \mathbf{G}, \ j \in \mathbf{N}_g, \ h \neq g \qquad (10)$$

$$\sum_{j \in N_g} u_{hgj} \leq \lfloor \alpha_{hg} n_g \rfloor, \qquad\qquad h, g \in \mathbf{G}, \ h \neq g \qquad\qquad (11)$$

$$-\infty < L_{hgj} < \infty, \ y_{gj} \geq 0, \ \lambda_{ih} \geq 0, u_{hgj} \in \{0, 1\}.$$

Constraint (7) defines the variable L_{hgj} as the value of the function L_h evaluated at x^{gj}. Therefore, the continuous variable y_{gj}, defined in constraint (8), represents $\max\{L_h(x^{gj}) : \ h = 0, ..., G\}$; and consequently, x^{gj} lies in region R_h if, and only if, $y_{gj} = L_{hgj}$. The binary variable u_{hgj} is used to indicate whether or not x^{gj} lies in region R_h; i.e., whether or not the jth entity from group g is allocated to group h. In particular, constraint (9), together with the objective, force u_{ggj} to be 1 if, and only if, the jth entity from group g is correctly allocated to group g; and constraints (10) and (11) ensure that at most $\lfloor \alpha_{hg} n_g \rfloor$ (i.e., the greatest integer less than or equal to $\alpha_{hg} n_g$) group g entities are allocated to group h, $h \neq g$. One caveat regarding the indicator variables u_{hgj} is that although the condition $u_{hgj} = 0$, $h \neq g$, implies (by constraint (10)) that $x^{gj} \notin R_h$, the converse need not hold. As a consequence, the number of misclassifications may be overcounted. However, in our preliminary numerical study we found that the actual amount of overcounting is minimal. For example, one could force the converse (thus, $u_{hgj} = 1$ if and only if $x^{gj} \in R_h$) by adding constraints $y_{gj} - L_{hgj} \leq M(1 - u_{hgj})$. Finally, we note that the parameters M and ε are extraneous to the discriminant analysis problem itself, but are needed in the model to control the indicator variables u_{hgj}. The intention is for M and ε to be, respectively, large and small positive constants.

3.3 Model variations

We explore different variations in the model to grasp the quality of the solution and the associated computational effort.

A first variation involves transforming Model 1 to an equivalent linear mixed integer model. In particular, Model 2 replaces the N constraints defined in (8) with the following system of $3GN + 2N$ constraints:

$$y_{gj} \geq L_{hgj}, \qquad\qquad h, g \in \mathbf{G}, \ j \in \mathbf{N}_g \qquad\qquad (12)$$

$$\tilde{y}_{hgj} - L_{hgj} \leq M(1 - v_{hgj}), \qquad h, g \in \mathbf{G}, \ j \in \mathbf{N}_g \qquad\qquad (13)$$

$$\tilde{y}_{hgj} \leq \hat{\pi}_h \hat{p}_h(x^{gj}) v_{hgj}, \qquad h, g \in \mathbf{G}, \ j \in \mathbf{N}_g \qquad\qquad (14)$$

$$\sum_{h \in G} v_{hgj} \leq 1, \qquad\qquad g \in \mathbf{G}, \ j \in \mathbf{N}_g \qquad\qquad (15)$$

$$\sum_{h \in G} \tilde{y}_{hgj} = y_{gj}, \qquad\qquad g \in \mathbf{G}, \ j \in \mathbf{N}_g \qquad\qquad (16)$$

where $\tilde{y}_{hgj} \geq 0$ and $v_{hgj} \in \{0, 1\}$, $h, g \in \mathbf{G}, j \in \mathbf{N}_g$. These constraints, together with the non-negativity of y_{gj} force $y_{gj} = \max\{0, L_{hgj} : h = 1, ..., G\}$.

The second variation involves transforming Model 1 to a heuristic linear MIP model. This is done by replacing the nonlinear constraint (8) with $y_{gj} \geq L_{hgj}$, $h, g \in \mathbf{G}, j \in \mathbf{N}_g$, and including penalty terms in the objective function. In particular, Model 3 has the objective

$$\max \sum_{g \in G} \sum_{j \in N_g} \beta u_{ggj} - \sum_{g \in G} \sum_{j \in N_g} \gamma y_{gj},$$

where β and γ are positive constants. This model is heuristic in that there is nothing to force $y_{gj} = \max\{0, L_{hgj} : h = 1, ..., G\}$. However, since in addition to trying to force as many u_{ggj}s to one as possible, the objective in Model 3 also tries to make the y_{gj}s as small as possible, and the optimizer tends to drive y_{gj} towards $\max\{0, L_{hgj} : h = 1, ..., G\}$. We remark that β and γ could be stratified by a group (i.e., introduce possibly distinct $\beta_g, \gamma_g, g \in \mathbf{G}$) to model the relative importance of certain groups to be correctly classified.

A reasonable modification to Models 1, 2 and 3 involves relaxing the constraints specified by (11). Rather than placing restrictions on the number of type g training entities classified into group h, for all $h, g \in \mathbf{G}, h \neq g$, one could simply place an upper bound on the *total* number of misclassified training entities. In this case, the $G(G-1)$ constraints specified by (11) would be replaced by the single constraint

$$\sum_{g \in G} \sum_{h \in G \setminus \{g\}} \sum_{j \in N_g} u_{hgj} \leq \lfloor \alpha N \rfloor \tag{17}$$

where α is a constant between 0 and 1. We will refer to Models 1, 2 and 3, modified in this way, as Models 1T, 2T and 3T, respectively. Of course, other modifications are also possible. For instance, one could place restrictions on the total number of type g points misclassified for each $g \in \mathbf{G}$. Thus, in place of the constraints specified in (17), one would include the constraints $\sum_{h \in G \setminus \{g\}} \sum_{j \in N_g} u_{hgj} \leq \lfloor \alpha_g N \rfloor$, $g \in \mathbf{G}$, where $0 < \alpha_g < 1$.

We also explore a heuristic linear model of Model 1. In particular, consider the linear program (DALP):

$$\max \sum_{g \in G} \sum_{j \in N_g} (c_1 w_{gj} + c_2 y_{gj}) \tag{18}$$

s.t.

$$L_{hgj} = \pi_h \hat{p}_h(x^{gj}) - \sum_{i \in G \setminus h} \lambda_{ih} \hat{p}_i(x^{gj}), \quad h, g \in \mathbf{G}, \ j \in \mathbf{N}_g \tag{19}$$

$$L_{ggj} - L_{hgj} + w_{gj} \geq 0, \quad h, g \in \mathbf{G}, \ h \neq g, \ j \in \mathbf{N}_g \tag{20}$$

$$L_{ggj} \quad + w_{gj} \geq 0, \quad g \in \mathbf{G}, \ j \in \mathbf{N}_g, \tag{21}$$

$$-L_{hgj} + y_{gj} \geq 0, \quad h, g \in \mathbf{G}, \ j \in \mathbf{N}_g, \tag{22}$$

$$-\infty < L_{hgj} < \infty, \ w_{gj}, \ y_{gj}, \ \lambda_{ih} \geq 0.$$

Constraint (19) defines the variable L_{hgj} as the value of the function L_h evaluated at x^{gj}. As the optimization solver searches through the set of feasible solutions, the λ_{ih} variables will vary, causing the L_{hgj} variables to assume different values. Constraints (20), (21) and (22) link the objective-function variables with the L_{hgj} variables in such a way that correct classification of training entities, and allocation of training entities into the reserved-judgment region, are captured by the objective-function variables. In particular, if the optimization solver drives w_{gj} to zero for some g,j pair, then constraints (20) and (21) imply that $L_{ggj} = \max\{0, L_{hgj} : h \in \mathbf{G}\}$. Hence, the jth entity from group g is correctly classified. If, on the other hand, the optimal solution yields $y_{gj} = 0$ for some g,j pair, then constraint (22) implies that $\max\{0, L_{hgj} : h \in \mathbf{G}\} = 0$. Thus, the jth entity from group g is placed in the reserved-judgment region. (Of course, it is possible for both w_{gj} and y_{gj} to be zero. One should decide prior to solving the linear program how to interpret the classification in such cases.) If both w_{gj} and y_{gj} are positive, the jth entity from group g is misclassified.

The optimal solution yields a set of λ_{ih}s that best allocates the training entities (i.e., "best" in terms of minimizing the penalty objective function). The optimal λ_{ih}s can then be used to define the functions L_h, $h \in G$, which in turn can be used to classify a new entity with feature vector $x \in \mathbb{R}^k$ by simply computing the index at which $\max\{L_h(x) : h \in \{0, 1, ..., G\}\}$ is achieved.

Note that Model DALP places no a priori bound on the number of misclassified training entities. However, since the objective is to minimize a weighted combination of the variables w_{gj} and y_{gj}, the optimizer will attempt to drive these variables to zero. Thus, the optimizer is, in essence, attempting either to correctly classify training entities ($w_{gj} = 0$), or to place them in the reserved-judgment region ($y_{gj} = 0$). By varying the weights c_1 and c_2, one has a means of controlling the optimizer's emphasis for correctly classifying training entities versus placing them in the reserved-judgment region. If $c_2/c_1 < 1$, the optimizer will tend to place a greater emphasis on driving the w_{gj} variables to zero than driving the y_{gj} variables to zero (conversely, if $c_2/c_1 > 1$). Hence, when $c_2/c_1 < 1$, one should expect to get relatively more entities correctly classified, fewer placed in the reserved-judgment region, and more misclassified, than when $c_2/c_1 > 1$. An extreme case is when $c_2 = 0$. In this case, there is no emphasis on driving y_{gj} to zero (the reserved-judgment region is thus ignored), and the full emphasis of the optimizer is on driving w_{gj} to zero.

Table 1 summarizes the number of constraints, the total number of variables, and the number of 0/1 variables in each of the discrete support vector machine models and in the heuristic LP model (DALP). Clearly, even for moderately-sized discriminant analysis problems, the MIP instances are relatively large. Also, note that Model 2 is larger than Model 3, both in terms of the number of constraints and the number of variables. However, it is important to keep in mind that the difficulty of solving an MIP problem cannot, in general, be predicted solely by its size; problem structure has a direct and substantial bearing on the effort required to find optimal solutions. The LP

Table 1. Model size.

Model	Type	Constraints	Total Variables	0/1 Variables
1	nonlinear MIP	$2GN + N + G(G-1)$	$2GN + N + G(G-1)$	GN
2	linear MIP	$5GN + 2N + G(G-1)$	$4GN + N + G(G-1)$	$2GN$
3	linear MIP	$3GN + G(G-1)$	$2GN + N + G(G-1)$	GN
1T	nonlinear MIP	$2GN + N + 1$	$2GN + N + G(G-1)$	GN
2T	linear MIP	$5GN + 2N + 1$	$4GN + N + G(G-1)$	$2GN$
3T	linear MIP	$3GN + 1$	$2GN + N + G(G-1)$	GN
DALP	linear program	$3GN$	$NG + N + G(G-1)$	0

relaxation of these MIP models pose computational challenges as commercial LP solvers return (optimal) LP solutions that are infeasible due to the equality constraints and the use of big M and small ε in the formulation.

It is interesting to note that the set of feasible solutions for Model 2 is "tighter" than that for Model 3. In particular, if F_i denotes the set of feasible solutions of Model i, then

$$F_1 = \{(L, \lambda, u, y) : \text{ there exists } \tilde{y}, v \text{ such that } (L, \lambda, u, y, \tilde{y}, v) \in F_2\} \subsetneq F_3. \tag{23}$$

Novelties of the classification models developed herein: 1) they are suitable for discriminant analysis given any number of groups, 2) they accept heterogeneous types of attributes as input, 3) they use a parametric approach to reduce high-dimensional attribute spaces, and 4) they allow constraints on the number of misclassifications and utilize a reserved judgment to facilitate the reduction of misclassifications. The latter point opens the possibility of performing multistage analyses.

Clearly, the advantage of an LP model over an MIP model is that the associated problem instances are computationally much easier to solve. However, the most important criterion in judging a method for obtaining discriminant rules is how the rules perform in correctly classifying new unseen entities. Once the rule is developed, applying it to a new entity to determine its group is trivial. Extensive computational experiments have been performed to gauge the qualities of solutions of different models [28, 49, 42, 43, 12, 13].

3.4 Computational strategies

The mixed integer programming models described herein offer a computational avenue for numerically estimating optimal values for the λ_{ih} parameters in Anderson's formulae. However, it should be emphasized that mixed integer programming problems are themselves difficult to solve. Anderson [1] himself noted the extreme difficulty of finding an optimal set of λ_{ih}s. Indeed,

MIP is an NP-hard problem (e.g., see [29]). Nevertheless, due to the fact that integer variables — and in particular, 0/1 variables — are a powerful modeling tool, a wide variety of real-world problems have been modeled as mixed integer programs. Consequently, much effort has been invested in developing computational strategies for solving MIP problem instances.

The numerical work reported in Section 4 is based on an MIP solver which is built on top of a general-purpose mixed integer research code, MIPSOL [38]. (A competitive commercial solver (CPLEX) was not effective in solving the problem instances considered.) The general-purpose code integrates state-of-the-art MIP computational devices such as problem preprocessing, primal heuristics, global and local reduced-cost fixing, and cutting planes into a branch-and-bound framework. The code has been shown to be effective in solving a wide variety of large-scale real-world instances [6]. For our MIP instances, special techniques such as variable aggregation, a heuristic branching scheme, and hypergraphic cut generations are employed [28, 21, 12].

4 Classification results on real-world applications

The main objective in discriminant analysis is to derive rules that can be used to classify entities into groups. Computationally, the challenge lies in the effort expended to develop such a rule. Once the rule is developed, applying it to a new entity to determine its group is trivial. Feasible solutions obtained from our classification models correspond to predictive rules. Empirical results [28, 49] indicate that the resulting classification model instances are computationally very challenging, and even intractable by competitive commercial MIP solvers. However, the resulting predictive rules prove to be very promising, offering correct classification rates on new unknown data ranging from 80% to 100% on various types of biological/medical problems. Our results indicate that the general-purpose classification framework that we have designed has the potential to be a very powerful predictive method for clinical settings.

The choice of mixed integer programming (MIP) as the underlying modeling and optimization technology for our support vector machine classification model is guided by the desire to simultaneously incorporate a variety of important and desirable properties of predictive models within a general framework. MIP itself allows for the incorporation of continuous and discrete variables and linear and nonlinear constraints, providing a flexible and powerful modeling environment.

4.1 Validation of model and computational effort

We performed ten-fold cross validation, and designed simulation and comparison studies on our preliminary models. The results, reported in [28, 49], show the methods are promising, based on applications to both simulated data and datasets from the machine learning database repository [62]. Furthermore, our methods compare well and at times superior to existing methods, such as artificial neural networks, quadratic discriminant analysis, tree classification, and other support vector machines, on real biological and medical data.

4.2 Applications to biological and medical problems

Our mathematical modeling and computational algorithm design shows great promise as the resulting predictive rules are able to produce higher rates of correct classification on new biological data (with unknown group status) compared to existing classification methods. This is partly due to the transformation of raw data via the set of constraints in (7). While most support vector machines [53] directly determine the hyperplanes of separation using raw data, our approach transforms the raw data via a probabilistic model, before the determination of the supporting hyperplanes. Further, the separation is driven by maximizing the sum of binary variables (representing correct or incorrect classification of entities), instead of maximizing the margin between groups, or minimizing a sum of errors (representing distances of entities from hyperplanes) as in other support vector machines. The combination of these two strategies offers better classification capability. Noise in the transformed data is not as profound as in raw data. And the magnitudes of the errors do not skew the determination of the separating hyperplanes, as all entities have *equal* importance when correct classification is being counted.

To highlight the broad applicability of our approach, in this paper we briefly summarize the application of our predictive models and solution algorithms to eight different biological problems. Each of the projects was carried out in close partnership with experimental biologists and/or clinicians. Applications to finance and other industry applications are described elsewhere [12, 28, 49].

Determining the type of Erythemato-Squamous disease

The differential diagnosis of erythemato-squamous diseases is an important problem in dermatology. They all share the clinical features of erythema and scaling, with very little differences. The six groups are psoriasis, seboreic dermatitis, lichen planus, pityriasis rosea, chronic dermatitis, and pityriasis rubra pilaris. Usually a biopsy is necessary for the diagnosis, but unfortunately these diseases share many histopathological features as well. Another difficulty for the differential diagnosis is that a disease may show the features of another disease at the beginning stage and may have the characteristic features at the following stages [62].

The six groups consist of 366 subjects (112,61,72,49,52,20 respectively) with 34 clinical attributes. Patients were first evaluated clinically with 12 features. Afterwards, skin samples were taken for the evaluation of 22 histopathological features. The values of the histopathological features are determined by an analysis of the samples under a microscope. The 34 attributes include 1) clinical attributes: erythema, scaling, definite borders, itching, koebner phenomenon, polygonal papules, follicular papules, oral mucosal involvement, knee and elbow involvement, scalp involvement, family history, age; and 2) histopathological attributes: melanin incontinence, eosinophils in the infiltrate, PNL infiltrate, fibrosis of the papillary dermis, exocytosis, acanthosis, hyperkeratosis, parakeratosis, clubbing of the rete ridges, elongation of the rete ridges, thinning of the suprapapillary epidermis, spongiform pustule, munro microabcess, focal hypergranulosis, disappearance of the granular layer, vacuolisation and damage of basal layer, spongiosis, saw-tooth appearance of retes, follicular horn plug, perifollicular parakeratosis, inflammatory monoluclear infiltrate, band-like infiltrate.

Our multi-group classification model selected 27 discriminatory attributes, and successfully classified the patients into six groups, each with an unbiased correct classification of greater than 93% (with 100% correct rate for groups 1, 3, 5, 6) with an average overall accuracy of 98%. Using 250 subjects to develop the rule, and testing the remaining 116 patients, we obtain a prediction accuracy of 91%.

Predicting aberrant CpG island methylation in human cancer [22, 23]

Epigenetic silencing associated with aberrant methylation of promoter region CpG islands is one mechanism leading to loss of the tumor suppressor function in human cancer. Profiling of CpG island methylation indicates that some genes are more frequently methylated than others, and that each tumor type is associated with a unique set of methylated genes. However, little is known about why certain genes succumb to this aberrant event. To address this question, we used Restriction Landmark Genome Scanning (RLGS) to analyze the susceptibility of 1749 unselected CpG islands to de novo methylation driven by overexpression of DNMT1. We found that, whereas the overall incidence of CpG island methylation increased in cells overexpressing DNMT1, not all loci were equally affected. The majority of CpG islands (69.9%) were resistant to de novo methylation, regardless of DNMT1 overexpression. In contrast, we identified a subset of methylation-prone CpG islands (3.8%) that were consistently hypermethylated in multiple DNMT1 overexpressing clones. Methylation-prone and methylation-resistant CpG islands were not significantly different with respect to size, C+G content, CpG frequency, chromosomal location, or gene- or promoter-association. To discriminate methylation-prone from methylation-resistant CpG islands, we developed a novel DNA pattern recognition model and algorithm [45], and coupled our predictive model described herein with the patterns found. We were able to derive a classification function based on the frequency of seven novel sequence patterns that was capable of discriminating methylation-prone from methylation-resistant CpG islands with 90% correctness upon cross-validation, and 85% accuracy when tested against blind CpG islands unknown to us on the methylation status. The data indicate that CpG islands differ in their intrinsic susceptibility to de novo methylation, and suggest that the propensity for a CpG island to become aberrantly methylated can be predicted based on its sequence context.

The significance of this research is two-fold. First, the identification of sequence patterns/attributes that distinguish methylation-prone CpG islands will lead to a better understanding of the basic mechanisms underlying aberrant CpG island methylation. Because genes that are silenced by methylation are otherwise structurally sound, the potential for reactivating these genes by blocking or reversing the methylation process represents an exciting new molecular target for chemotherapeutic intervention. A better understanding of the factors that contribute to aberrant methylation, including the identification of sequence elements that may act to target aberrant methylation, will be an important step in achieving this long-term goal. Secondly, the classification of the more than 29,000 known (but as yet unclassified) CpG islands in human chromosomes will provide an important resource for the identification of novel gene targets for further study as potential molecular markers that could impact both cancer prevention and treatment. Extensive RLGS fingerprint information (and thus potential training sets of methylated CpG islands) already exists for a number of human tumor types, including breast, brain, lung, leukemias, hepatocellular carcinomas, and PNET [17, 18, 26, 67]. Thus, the methods and tools developed are directly applicable to CpG island methylation data derived from human tumors. Moreover, new microarray-based techniques capable of 'profiling' more than 7000 CpG islands have been developed and applied to human breast cancers [9, 74, 75]. We are uniquely poised to take advantage of the tumor CpG island methylation profile information that will likely be generated using these techniques over the next several years. Thus, our general-predictive modeling framework has the potential to lead to improved diagnosis and prognosis and treatment planning for cancer patients.

Discriminant analysis of cell motility and morphology data in human lung carcinoma [14]

This study focuses on the differential effects of extracellular matrix proteins on the motility and morphology of human lung epidermoid carcinoma cells. The behavior of carcinoma cells is contrasted with that of normal L-132 cells, resulting in a method for the prediction of metastatic potential. Data collected from time-lapsed videomicroscopy were used to simultaneously produce quantitative measures of motility and morphology. The data were subsequently analyzed using our discriminant analysis model and algorithm to discover relationships between motility, morphology, and substratum. Our discriminant analysis tools enabled the consideration of many more cell attributes than is customary in cell motility studies. The observations correlate with behaviors seen in vivo and suggest specific roles for the extracellular matrix proteins and their integrin receptors in metastasis. Cell translocation in vitro has been associated with malignancy, as has an elongated phenotype [76] and a rounded phenotype [66]. Our study suggests that extracellular matrix proteins contribute in different ways to the malignancy of cancer cells, and that multiple malignant phenotypes exist.

Ultrasonic assisted cell disruption for drug delivery [48]

Although biological effects of ultrasounds must be avoided for safe diagnostic applications, an ultrasound's ability to disrupt cell membranes has attracted interest in it as a method to facilitate drug and gene delivery. This preliminary study seeks to develop rules for predicting the degree of cell membrane disruption based on specified ultrasound parameters and measured acoustic signals. Too much ultrasound destroys cells, while cell membranes will not open up for absorption of macromolecules when too little ultrasound is applied. The key is to increase cell permeability to allow absorption of macromolecules, and to apply ultrasound transiently to disrupt viable cells so as to enable exogenous material to enter without cell damage. Thus our task is to uncover a "predictive rule" of ultrasound-mediated disruption of red blood cells using acoustic spectrums and measurements of cell permeability recorded in experiments.

Our predictive model and solver for generating prediction rules are applied to data obtained from a sequence of experiments on bovine red blood cells. For each experiment, the attributes consist of 4 ultrasound parameters, acoustic measurements at 400 frequencies, and a measure of cell membrane disruption. To avoid over-training, various feature combinations of the 404 predictor variables are selected when developing the classification rule. The results indicate that the variable combination consisting of ultrasound exposure time and acoustic signals measured at the driving frequency and its higher harmonics yields the best rule. Our method compares favorably with the classification tree and other ad hoc approaches, with a correct classification rate of 80% upon cross-validation and 85% when classifying new unknown entities. Our methods used for deriving the prediction rules are broadly applicable, and could be used to develop prediction rules in other scenarios involving different cell types or tissues. These rules and the methods used to derive them could be used for real-time feedback about ultrasound's biological effects. For example, it could assist clinicians during a drug delivery process, or could be imported into an implantable device inside the body for automatic drug delivery and monitoring.

Identification of tumor shape and volume in treatment of sarcoma [46]

This project involves the determination of tumor shape for adjuvant brachytherapy treatment of sarcoma, based on catheter images taken after surgery. In this application, the entities are overlapping consecutive triplets of catheter markings, each of which is used for determining the shape of the tumor contour. The triplets are to be classified into one of two groups: Group 1 = [triplets for which the middle catheter marking should be bypassed], and Group 2 = [triplets for which the middle marking should not be bypassed]. To develop and validate a classification rule, we used clinical data collected from fifteen soft tissue sarcoma (STS) patients. Cumulatively, this comprised 620 triplets of catheter markings. By careful (and tedious) clinical analysis of the geometry of these triplets, 65 were determined to belong to Group 1, the "bypass" group, and 555 were determined to belong to Group 2, the "do-not-bypass" group.

A set of measurements associated with each triplet is then determined. The choice of what attributes to measure to best distinguish triplets as belonging to Group 1 or Group 2 is non trivial. The attributes involved distance between each pair of markings, angles, and curvature formed by the three triplet markings. Based on the selected attributes, our predictive model was used to develop a classification rule. The resulting rule provides 98% correct classification on cross-validation, and was capable of correctly determining/predicting 95% of the shape of the tumor on new patients' data. We remark that the current clinical procedure requires manual outline based on markers in films of the tumor volume. This study was the first to use automatic construction of tumor shape for sarcoma adjuvant brachytherapy [46, 47].

Discriminant analysis of biomarkers for prediction of early atherosclerosis [44]

Oxidative stress is an important etiologic factor in the pathogenesis of vascular disease. Oxidative stress results from an imbalance between injurious oxidant and protective antioxidant events in which the former predominate [59, 68]. This results in the modification of proteins and DNA, alteration in gene expression, promotion of inflammation, and deterioration in endothelial function in the vessel wall, all processes that ultimately trigger or exacerbate the atherosclerotic process [16, 72]. It was hypothesized that novel biomarkers of oxidative stress would predict early atherosclerosis in a relatively healthy non-smoking population who are free from cardiovascular disease. One hundred and twenty seven healthy non-smokers, without known clinical atherosclerosis had carotid intima media thickness (IMT) measured using ultrasound. Plasma oxidative stress was estimated by measuring plasma lipid hydroperoxides using the determination of reactive oxygen metabolites (d-ROMs) test. Clinical measurements include traditional risk factors such as age, sex, low density lipoprotein (LDL), high density lipoprotein (HDL), triglycerides, cholesterol, body-mass-index (BMI), hypertension, diabetes mellitus, smoking history, family history of CAD, Framingham risk score, and Hs-CRP.

For this prediction, the patients are first clustered into two groups: (Group 1: IMT $>= 0.68$, Group 2: IMT < 0.68). Based on this separator, 30 patients belong to Group 1 and 97 belong to Group 2. Through each iteration, the classification method trains and learns from the input training set and returns the most discriminatory patterns among the 14 clinical measurements; ultimately resulting in the development of a prediction rule based on observed values of these discriminatory patterns among the patient data. Using all 127 patients as a training set, the predictive model identified age, sex, BMI, HDLc, Fhx CAD < 60, hs-CRP and d-ROM as discriminatory attributes that together provide unbiased correct classification of 90% and 93%, respectively, for Group 1 (IMT >= 0.68) and Group 2 (IMT < 0.68) patients. To further test the power of the classification method for correctly predicting the IMT status on new/unseen patients, we randomly selected a smaller patient training set of size 90. The predictive rule from this training set yields 80% and 89% correct rates for predicting the remaining 37 patients into Group 1 and Group 2, respectively. The importance of d-ROM as a discriminatory predictor for IMT status was confirmed during the machine learning process. This biomarker was selected in every iteration as the "machine" learned and trained to develop a predictive rule to correctly classify patients in the training set. We also performed predictive analysis using Framingham Risk Score and d-ROM; in this case the unbiased correct classification rates (for the 127 individuals) for Groups 1 and 2 are 77% and 84%, respectively. This is the first study to illustrate that this measure of oxidative stress can be effectively used along with traditional risk factors to generate a predictive rule that can potentially serve as an inexpensive clinical diagnostic tool for the prediction of early atherosclerosis.

Fingerprinting native and angiogenic microvascular networks through pattern recognition and discriminant analysis of functional perfusion data [50]

The cardiovascular system provides oxygen and nutrients to the entire body. Pathological conditions that impair normal microvascular perfusion can result in tissue ischemia, with potentially serious clinical effects. Conversely, development of new vascular structures fuels the progression of cancer, macular degeneration and atherosclerosis. Fluorescence-microangiography offers superb imaging of the functional perfusion of new and existent microvasculature, but quantitative analysis of the complex capillary patterns is challenging. We developed an automated pattern-recognition algorithm to systematically analyze the microvascular networks, and then apply our classification model herein to generate a predictive rule. The pattern-recognition algorithm identifies the complex vascular branching patterns, and the predictive rule demonstrates 100% and 91% correct classification on perturbed (diseased) and normal tissue perfusion, respectively. We confirmed that transplantation of normal bone marrow to mice in which genetic deficiency resulted in impaired angiogenesis eliminated predicted differences and restored normal-tissue perfusion patterns (with 100% correctness). The pattern recognition and classification method offers an elegant solution for the automated fingerprinting of microvascular networks that could contribute to better understanding of angiogenic mechanisms and be utilized to diagnose and monitor microvascular deficiencies. Such information would be valuable for early detection and monitoring of functional abnormalities before they produce obvious and lasting effects, which may include improper perfusion of tissue, or support of tumor development.

The algorithm can be used to discriminate between the angiogenic response in a native healthy specimen compared to groups with impairment due to age, chemical or other genetic deficiency. Similarly, it can be applied to analyze angiogenic responses as a result of various treatments. This will serve two important goals. First, the identification of discriminatory patterns/attributes that distinguish angiogenesis status will lead to a better understanding of the basic mechanisms underlying this process. Because therapeutic control of angiogenesis could influence physiological and pathological processes such as wound and tissue repairing, cancer progression and metastasis, or macular degeneration, the ability to understand it under different conditions will offer new insight in developing novel therapeutic interventions, monitoring and treatment, especially in aging, and heart disease. Thus, our study and the results form the foundation of a valuable diagnostic tool for changes in the functionality of the microvasculature and for discovery of drugs that alter the angiogenic response. The methods can be applied to tumor diagnosis, monitoring and prognosis. In particular, it will be possible to derive microangiographic fingerprints to acquire specific microvascular patterns associated with early stages of tumor development. Such "angioprinting" could become an extremely helpful early diagnostic modality, especially for easily accessible tumors such as skin cancer.

Prediction of protein localization sites

The protein localization database consists of 8 groups with a total of 336 instances (143, 77, 52, 35, 20, 5, 2, 2, respectively) with 7 attributes [62]. The eight groups are eight localization sites of protein, including cp (cytoplasm), im (inner membrane without signal sequence), pp (perisplasm), imU (inner membrane, uncleavable signal sequence), om (outer membrane), omL (outer membrane lipoprotein), imL (inner membrane lipoprotein), and imS (inner membrane, cleavable signal sequence). However, the last four groups are taken out from our classification experiment since the population sizes are too small to ensure significance.

The seven attributes include mcg (McGeoch's method for signal sequence recognition), gvh (von Heijne's method for signal sequence recognition), lip (von Heijne's Signal Peptidase II consensus sequence score), chg (Presence of charge on N-terminus of predicted lipoproteins), aac (score of discriminant analysis of the amino acid content of outer membrane and periplasmic proteins), alm1 (score of the ALOM membrane spanning region prediction program), and alm2 (score of ALOM program after excluding putative cleavable signal regions from the sequence).

In the classification we use 4 groups, 307 instances, with 7 attributes. Our classification model selected the discriminatory patterns mcg, gvh, alm1, and alm2 to form the predictive rule with unbiased correct classification rates of 89%, compared to the results of 81% by other classification models [36].

5 Summary and conclusion

In the article, we present a class of general-purpose predictive models that we have developed based on the technology of large-scale optimization and support-vector machines [28, 49, 42, 43, 12, 13]. Our models seek to maximize the correct classification rate while constraining the number of misclassifications in each group. The models incorporate the following features: 1) the ability to classify any number of distinct groups; 2) allowing incorporation of heterogeneous types of attributes as input; 3) a high-dimensional data transformation that eliminates noise and errors in biological data; 4) constraining the misclassification in each group and a reserved-judgment region that provides a safeguard against over-training (which tends to lead to high misclassification rates from the resulting predictive rule); and 5) successive multi-stage classification capability to handle data points placed in the reserved-judgment region. The performance and predictive power of the classification models is validated through a broad class of biological and medical applications.

Classification models are critical to medical advances as they can be used in genomic, cell, molecular, and system level analyses to assist in early prediction, diagnosis and detection of disease, as well as for intervention and monitoring. As shown in the CpG island study for human cancer, such prediction and diagnosis opens up novel therapeutic sites for early intervention. The ultrasound application illustrates its application to a novel drug delivery mechanism, assisting clinicians during a drug delivery process, or in devising implantable devices into the body for automated drug delivery and monitoring. The lung cancer cell motility offers an understanding of how cancer cells behave under different protein media, thus assisting in the identification of potential gene therapy and target treatment. Prediction of the shape of a cancer tumor bed provides a personalized treatment design, replacing manual estimates by sophisticated computer predictive models. Prediction of early atherosclerosis through inexpensive biomarker measurements and traditional risk factors can serve as a potential clinical diagnostic tool for routine physical and health maintenance, alerting doctors and patients to the need for early intervention to prevent serious vascular disease. Fingerprinting of microvascular networks opens up the possibility of early diagnosis of perturbed systems in the body that may trigger disease (e.g., genetic deficiency, diabetes, aging, obesity, macular degeneracy, tumor formation), identifying the target site for treatment, and monitoring the prognosis and success of treatment. Thus, classification models serve as a basis for predictive medicine where the desire is to diagnose early and provide personalized target intervention. This has the potential to reduce healthcare costs, improve the success of treatment and quality-of-life of patients.

In [11], we have showed that our multi-category constrained discrimination analysis predictive model is strongly universally consistent. Further theoretical studys will be performed on these models to understand their characteristics and the sensitivity of the predictive patterns to model/parameter variations. The modeling framework for discrete support vector machines offers great flexibility, enabling one to simultaneously incorporate the features as listed above, as well as many other features. However, deriving the predictive rules for such problems can be computationally demanding, due to the NP-hard nature of mixed integer programming [29]. We continue to work on improving optimization algorithms utilizing novel cutting plane and branch-and-bound strategies, fast heuristic algorithms, and parallel algorithms [6, 21, 38–41, 51, 52].

Acknowledgement

This research was partially supported by the National Science Foundation.

References

1. J. A. Anderson. Constrained discrimination between k populations. *Journal of the Royal Statistical Society, Series B*, 31:123–139, 1969.
2. S. M. Bajgier and A. V. Hill. An experimental comparison of statistical and linear programming approaches to the discriminant problems. *Decision Sciences*, 13:604–618, 1982.
3. K. P. Bennett and E. J. Bredensteiner. A parametric optimization method for machine learning. *INFORMS Journal on Computing*, 9:311–318, 1997.
4. K. P. Bennett and O. L. Mangasarian. Multicategory discrimination via linear programming. *Optimization Methods and Software*, 3:27–39, 1993.
5. C. M. Bishop. *Neural Networks for Pattern Recognition.* Oxford University Press, Oxford, 1995.
6. R. E. Bixby, W. Cook, A. Cox, and E. K. Lee. Computational experience with parallel mixed integer programming in a distributed environment. *Annals of Operations Research, Special Issue on Parallel Optimization*, 90:19–43, 1999.
7. P. S. Bradley, U. M. Fayyad, and O. L. Mangasarian. Mathematical programming for data mining: Formulations and challenges. *INFORMS Journal on Computing*, 11:217–238, 1999.
8. J. Breiman, R. Friedman, A. Olshen, and C. J. Stone. *Wadsworth & Brooks/Cole Advanced Books & Software*, Pacific Grove, CA, 1984.
9. G. J. Brock, T. H. Huang, C. M. Chen, and K. J. Johnson. A novel technique for the identification of CpG islands exhibiting altered methylation patterns (ICEAMP). *Nucleic Acids Research*, 29, 2001.
10. J. D. Broffit, R. H. Randles, and R. V. Hogg. Distribution-free partial discriminant analysis. *Journal of the American Statistical Association*, 71:934–939, 1976.

11. J. P. Brooks and E. K. Lee. Analysis of the consistency of a mixed integer programming-based multi-category constrained discriminant model. *Annals of Operations Research – Data Mining*. Submitted, 2006.

12. J. P. Brooks and E. K. Lee. Solving a mixed-integer programming formulation of a multi-category constrained discrimination model. *Proceedings of the 2006 INFORMS Workshop on Artificial Intelligence and Data Mining*, Pittsburgh, PA, Nov 2006.

13. J. P. Brooks and E. K. Lee. Mixed integer programming constrained discrimination model for credit screening. *Proceedings of the 2007 Spring Simulation Multiconference, Business and Industry Symposium*, Norfolk, VA, March 2007. ACM Digital Library, pages 1–6.

14. J. P. Brooks, Adele Wright, C. Zhu, and E. K. Lee. Discriminant analysis of motility and morphology data from human lung carcinoma cells placed on purified extracellular matrix proteins. *Annals of Biomedical Engineering*, in review, 2006.

15. T. M. Cavalier, J. P. Ignizio, and A. L. Soyster. Discriminant analysis via mathematical programming: certain problems and their causes. *Computers and Operations Research*, 16:353–362, 1989.

16. M. Chevion, E. Berenshtein, and E. R. Stadtman. Human studies related to protein oxidation: protein carbonyl content as a marker of damage. *Free Radical Research*, 33:S99–S108, 2000.

17. J. F. Costello, M. C. Fruhwald, D. J. Smiraglia, L. J. Rush, G. P. Robertson, X. Gao, F. A. Wright, J. D. Feramisco, P. Peltomaki, J. C. Lang, D. E. Schuller, L. Yu, C. D. Bloomfield, M. A. Caligiuri, A. Yates, R. Nishikawa, H. H. Su, N. J. Petrelli, X. Zhang, M. S. O'Dorisio, W. A. Held, W. K. Cavenee, and C. Plass. Aberrant CpG-island methylation has non-random and tumour-type-specific patterns. *Nature Genetics*, 24:132–138, 2000.

18. J. F. Costello, C. Plass, and W. K. Cavenee. Aberrant methylation of genes in low-grade astrocytomas. *Brain Tumor Pathology*, 17:49–56, 2000.

19. N. Cristianini and J. Shawe-Taylor. *An Introduction to Support Vector Machines and other kernel-based learning methods*. Cambridge University Press, 2000.

20. R. O. Duda, P. E. Hart, and D. G. Stork. *Pattern classification*. Wiley, 2nd edition, New York, 2001.

21. T. Easton, K. Hooker, and E. K. Lee. Facets of the independent set polytope. *Mathematical Programming B*, 98:177–199, 2003.

22. F. A. Feltus, E. K. Lee, J. F. Costello, C. Plass, and P. M. Vertino. Predicting aberrant CpG island methylation. *Proceedings of the National Academy of Sciences*, 100:12253–12258, 2003.

23. F. A. Feltus, E. K. Lee, J. F. Costello, C. Plass, and P. M. Vertino. DNA signatures associated with CpG island methylation states. *Genomics*, 87:572–579, 2006.

24. N. Freed and F. Glover. A linear programming approach to the discriminant problem. *Decision Sciences*, 12:68–74, 1981.

25. N. Freed and F. Glover. Evaluating alternative linear programming models to solve the two-group discriminant problem. *Decision Sciences*, 17:151–162, 1986.

26. M. C. Fruhwald, M. S. O'Dorisio, L. J. Rush, J. L. Reiter, D. J. Smiraglia, G. Wenger, J. F. Costello, P. S. White, R. Krahe, G. M. Brodeur, and C. Plass.

Gene amplification in NETs/medulloblastomas: mapping of a novel amplified gene within the MYCN amplicon. *Journal of Medical Genetics*, 37:501–509, 2000.

27. R. J. Gallagher, E. K. Lee, and D. Patterson. An optimization model for constrained discriminant analysis and numerical experiments with iris, thyroid, and heart disease datasets. in: Cimino jj. In *Proceedings of the 1996 American Medical Informatics Association*, pages 209–213, 1996.

28. R. J. Gallagher, E. K. Lee, and D.A. Patterson. Constrained discriminant analysis via 0/1 mixed integer programming. *Annals of Operations Research, Special Issue on Non-Traditional Approaches to Statistical Classification and Regression*, 74:65–88, 1997.

29. M. R. Garey and D. S. Johnson. *Computers and Intractability: A Guide to the Theory of NP-Completeness*. Freeman, New York, 1979.

30. W. V. Gehrlein. General mathematical programming formulations for the statistical classification problem. *Operations Research Letters*, 5:299–304, 1986.

31. M. P. Gessaman and P.H. Gessaman. A comparison of some multivariate discrimination procedures. *Journal of the American Statistical Association*, 67:468–472, 1972.

32. F. Glover. Improved linear programming models for discriminant analysis. *Decision Sciences*, 21:771–785, 1990.

33. F. Glover, S. Keene, and B. Duea. A new class of models for the discriminant problem. *Decision Sciences*, 19:269–280, 1988.

34. W. Gochet, A. Stam, V. Srinivasan, and S. Chen. Multigroup discriminant analysis using linear programming. *Operations Research*, 45:213–225, 1997.

35. J. D. F. Habbema, J. Hermans, and A. T. Van Der Burgt. Cases of doubt in allocation problems. *Biometrika*, 61:313–324, 1974.

36. P. Horton and K. Nakai. A probablistic classification system for predicting the cellular localization sites of proteins. *Intelligent Systems in Molecular Biology*, pages 109–115, 1996. St. Louis, United States.

37. G. J. Koehler and S. S. Erenguc. Minimizing misclassifications in linear discriminant analysis. *Decision Sciences*, 21:63–85, 1990.

38. E. K. Lee. Computational experience with a general purpose mixed 0/1 integer programming solver (MIPSOL). Software report, School of Industrial and Systems Engineering, Georgia Institute of Technology, 1997.

39. E. K. Lee. A linear-programming based parallel cutting plane algorithm for mixed integer programming problems. *Proceedings for the Third Scandinavian Workshop on Linear Programming*, pages 22–31, 1999.

40. E. K. Lee. Branch-and-bound methods. In Mauricio G. C. Resende and Panos M. Pardalos, editors, *Handbook of Applied Optimization*. Oxford University Press, 2001.

41. E. K. Lee. Generating cutting planes for mixed integer programming problems in a parallel distributed memory environment. *INFORMS Journal on Computing*, 16:1–28, 2004.

42. E. K. Lee. Discriminant analysis and predictive models in medicine. In S. J. Deng, editor, *Interdisciplinary Research in Management Science, Finance, and HealthCare*. Peking University Press, 2006. To appear.

43. E. K. Lee. Large-scale optimization-based classification models in medicine and biology. *Annals of Biomedical Engineering, Systems Biology and Bioinformatics*, 35:1095–1109, 2007.

44. E. K. Lee, S. Ashfaq, D. P. Jones, S. D. Rhodes, W. S. Weintrau, C. H. Hopper, V. Vaccarino, D. G. Harrison, and A. A. Quyyumi. Prediction of early atherosclerosis in healthy adults via novel markers of oxidative stress and d-roms. Working Paper, 2007.

45. E. K. Lee, T. Easton, and K. Gupta. Novel evolutionary models and applications to sequence alignment problems. *Operations Research in Medicine – Computing and Optimization in Medicine and Life Sciences*, 148:167–187, 2006.

46. E. K. Lee, A. Y. C. Fung, J. P. Brooks, and M. Zaider. Automated tumor volume contouring in soft-tissue sarcoma adjuvant brachytherapy treatment. *International Journal of Radiation Oncology, Biology and Physics*, 47:1891–1910, 2002.

47. E. K. Lee, A. Y. C. Fung, and M. Zaider. Automated planning volume contouring in soft-tissue sarcoma adjuvant brachytherapy treatment. *International Journal of Radiation Oncology Biology Physics*, 51, 2001.

48. E. K. Lee, R. Gallagher, A. Campbell, and M. Prausnitz. Prediction of ultrasound-mediated disruption of cell membranes using machine learning techniques and statistical analysis of acoustic spectra. *IEEE Transactions on Biomedical Engineering*, 51:1–9, 2004.

49. E. K. Lee, R. J. Gallagher, and D. Patterson. A linear programming approach to discriminant analysis with a reserved judgment region. *INFORMS Journal on Computing*, 15:23–41, 2003.

50. E. K. Lee, S. Jagannathan, C. Johnson, and Z. S. Galis. Fingerprinting native and angiogenic microvascular networks through pattern recognition and discriminant analysis of functional perfusion data. Submitted, 2006.

51. E. K. Lee and S. Maheshwary. Facets of conflict hypergraphs. Submitted to Mathematics of Operations Research, 2005.

52. E. K. Lee and J. Mitchell. Computational experience of an interior-point SQP algorithm in a parallel branch-and-bound framework. In J. Franks, J. Roos, J. Terlaky, and J. Zhang, editors, *High Performance Optimization Techniques*, pages 329–347. Kluwer Academic Publishers, 1997.

53. E. K. Lee and T. L. Wu. Classification and disease prediction via mathematical programming. In O. Seref, O. Kundakcioglu, and P. Pardalos, editors, *Data Mining, Systems Analysis, and Optimization in Biomedicine*, AIP Conference Proceedings, 953: 1–42, 2007.

54. J. M. Liittschwager and C. Wang. Integer programming solution of a classification problem. *Management Science*, 24:1515–1525, 1978.

55. T. S. Lim, W. Y. Loh, and Y. S. Shih. A comparison of prediction accuracy, complexity, and training time of thirty-three old and new classification algorithms. *Machine Learning*, 40:203–228, 2000.

56. O. L. Mangasarian. Mathematical programming in neural networks. *ORSA Journal on Computing*, 5:349–360, 1993.

57. O. L. Mangasarian. Mathematical programming in data mining. *Data Mining and Knowledge Discovery*, 1:183–201, 1997.

58. O. L. Mangasarian, W. N. Street, and W. H. Wolberg. Breast cancer diagnosis and prognosis via linear programming. *Operations Research*, 43:570–577, 1995.

59. J. M. McCord. The evolution of free radicals and oxidative stress. *The American Journal of Medicine*, 108:652–659, 2000.

60. G. J. McLachlan. *Discriminant Analysis and Statistical Pattern Recognition*. Wiley, New York, 1992.

61. K. R. Müller, S. Mika, G. Rätsch, K. Tsuda, and B. Schólkopf. An introduction to kernel-based learning algorithms. *IEEE Transactions on Neural Networks*, 12:181–201, 2001.

62. P. M. Murphy and D. W. Aha. UCI repository of machine learning databases. Technical report, Department of Information and Computer Science, University of California, Irvine, California, 1994.

63. T.-H. Ng and R. H. Randles. Distribution-free partial discrimination procedures. *Computers and Mathematics with Applications*, 12A:225–234, 1986.

64. R. Pavur and C. Loucopoulos. Examining optimal criterion weights in mixed integer programming approaches to the multiple-group classification problem. *Journal of the Operational Research Society*, 46:626–640, 1995.

65. C. P. Quesenberry and M. P. Gessaman. Nonparametric discrimination using tolerance regions. *Annals of Mathematical Statistics*, 39:664–673, 1968.

66. A. Raz and A. Ben-Zéev. Cell-contact and -architecture of malignant cells and their relationship to metastasis. *Cancer and Metastasis Reviews*, 6:3–21, 1987.

67. L. J. Rush, Z. Dai, D. J. Smiraglia, X. Gao, F. A. Wright, M. Fruhwald, J. F. Costello, W. A. Held, L. Yu, R. Krahe, J. E. Kolitz, C. D. Bloomfield, M. A. Caligiuri, and C. Plass. Novel methylation targets in de novo acute myeloid leukemia with prevalence of chromosome 11 loci. *Blood*, 97:3226–3233, 2001.

68. H. Sies. Oxidative stress: introductory comments. H. Sies, Editor, Oxidative stress, Academic Press, London, 1–8, 1985.

69. A. Stam. Nontraditional approaches to statistical classification: Some perspectives on Lp-norm methods. *Annals of Operations Research*, 74:1–36, 1997.

70. A. Stam and E. A. Joachimsthaler. Solving the classification problem in discriminant analysis via linear and nonlinear programming. *Decision Sciences*, 20:285–293, 1989.

71. A. Stam and C. T. Ragsdale. On the classification gap in mathematical-programming-based approaches to the discriminant problem. *Naval Research Logistics*, 39:545–559, 1992.

72. S. Tahara, M. Matsuo, and T. Kaneko. Age-related changes in oxidative damage to lipids and DNA in rat skin. *Mechanisms of Ageing and Development*, 122:415–426, 2001.

73. V. Vapnik. *The Nature of Statistical Learning Theory*. Springer-Verlag, 1999.

74. P. S. Yan, C. M. Chen, H. Shi, F. Rahmatpanah, S. H. Wei, C. W. Caldwell, and T. H. Huang. Dissecting complex epigenetic alterations in breast cancer using CpG island microarrays. *Cancer Research*, 61:8375–8380, 2001.

75. P. S. Yan, M. R. Perry, D. E. Laux, A. L. Asare, C. W. Caldwell, and T. H. Huang. CpG island arrays: an application toward deciphering epigenetic signatures of breast cancer. *Clinical Cancer Research*, 6:1432–1438, 2000.

76. A. Zimmermann and H. U. Keller. Locomotion of tumor cells as an element of invasion and metastasis. *Biomedicine & Pharmacotherapy*, 41:337–344, 1987.

77. C. Zopounidis and M. Doumpos. Multicriteria classification and sorting methods: A literature review. *European Journal of Operational Research*, 138:229–246, 2002.

Optimal reconstruction kernels in medical imaging

Alfred K. Louis

Department of Mathematics, Saarland University, 66041 Saarbrücken Germany
louis@num.uni-sb.de

Summary. In this paper we present techniques for deriving inversion algorithms in medical imaging. To this end we present a few imaging technologies and their mathematical models. They essentially consist of integral operators. The reconstruction is then recognized as the solution of an inverse problem. General strategies, the so-called approximate inverse, for deriving a solution are adapted. Results from real data are presented.

Keywords: 3D-Tomography, optimal algorithms (accuracy, efficiency, noise reduction), error bounds for influence of data noise, approximate inverse.

1 Introduction

The task in medical imaging is to provide, in a non-invasive way, information about the internal structure of the human body. The basic principle is that the patient is scanned by applying some sort of radiation and its interaction with the body is measured. This result is the data whose origin has to be identified. Hence we face an inverse problem.

There are several different imaging techniques and also different ways to characterize them. For the patient, a very substantial difference is whether the source is inside or outside the body, whether we have *emission* or *transmission* tomography.

From the diagnostic point of view the resulting information is a way to distinguish the different techniques. Some methods provide information about the density of the tissue as x-ray computer tomography, ultrasound computer tomography, or diffuse tomography. A distinction between properties of the tissues is possible with magnetic resonance imaging and impedance computer tomography. Finally the localization of activities is possible with biomagnetism, (electrical activities), and emission computer tomography, (nuclear activities of injected pharmaceuticals).

From a physical point of view the applied wavelengths can serve as a classification. The penetration of electromagnetic waves into the body is sufficient only for wavelengths smaller than $10^{-11}m$ or larger than a few cm respectively. In the extremely short ranges are x rays, single particle emission tomography and positron emission computer tomography. MRI uses wavelengths larger than $1m$; extremely long waves are used in biomagnetism. In the range of a few mm to a few cm are microwaves, ultrasound and light.

In this paper we present some principles in designing inversion algorithms in tomography. We concentrate on linear problems arising in connection with the Radon and the x-ray transform. In the original 2D x-ray CT problem, the Radon transform served as a mathematical model. Here one integrates over lines and the problem is to recover a function from its line integrals. The same holds in the 3D x-ray case, but in 3D the Radon transform integrates over planes, in general over $N-1$ - dimensional hyperplanes in $\mathbb{R}^N$. Hence here the so-called x-ray transform is the mathematical model. Further differences are in the parametrization of the lines. The 3D - Radon transform merely appears as a tool to derive inversion formula. In the early days of MRI (magnetic resonance imaging), in those days called NMR, nuclear magnetic resonance, it served as a mathematical model, see for example Marr-Chen-Lauterbur [26]. But then, due to the limitations of computer power in those days one changed the measuring procedure and scanned the Fourier transform of the searched-for function in two dimensions. The Radon transform has reappeared, now in three and even four dimensions as a mathematical model in EPRI (electron parametric resonance imaging) where spectral-spatial information is the goal, see, e.g., Kuppusamy et al. [11]. Here also incomplete data problems play a central role, see e.g. [12, 23].

The paper is organized as follows. We start with a general principle for reconstruction information from measured data, the so-called approximate inverse, see [16, 20]. The well-known inversion of the Radon transform is considered a model case for inversion. Finally, we consider a 3D x-ray problem and present reconstructions from real data.

2 Approximate inverse as a tool for deriving inversion algorithms

The integral operators appearing in medical imaging are typically compact operators between suitable Hilbert spaces. The inverse operator of those compact operators with infinite dimensional range are not continuous, which means that the unavoidable data errors are amplified in the solution. Hence one has to be very careful in designing inversion algorithms has to balance the demand for highest possible accuracy and the necessary damping of the influence of unavoidable data errors. From the theoretical point of view, exact inversion formulae are nice, but they do not take care of data errors. The way out of this dilemma is the use of approximate inversion formulas whose principles are explained in the following.

For approximating the solution of

$$Af = g$$

we apply the method of approximate inverse, see [16]. The basic idea works as follows: choose a so-called mollifier $e_\gamma(x, y)$ which, for a fixed reconstruction point x, is a function of the variable y and which approximates the delta distribution for the point x. The parameter γ acts as regularization parameter. Simply think in the case of one spatial variable x of

$$e_\gamma(x, y) = \frac{1}{2\gamma}\chi_{[x-\gamma, x+\gamma]}(y)$$

where χ_Ω denotes the characteristic function of Ω. Then the mollifier fulfills

$$\int e_\gamma(x, y)dy = 1 \tag{1}$$

for all x and the function

$$f_\gamma(x) = \int f(y)e_\gamma(x, y)dy$$

converges for $\gamma \to 0$ to f. The larger the parameter γ, the larger the interval where the averaging takes place, and hence the stronger the smoothing. Now solve for fixed reconstruction point x the auxiliary problem

$$A^*\psi_\gamma(x, \cdot) = e_\gamma(x, \cdot) \tag{2}$$

where $e_\gamma(x, \cdot)$ is the chosen approximation to the delta distribution for the point x, and put

$$\begin{aligned} f_\gamma(x) &= \langle f, e_\gamma(x, \cdot)\rangle \\ &= \langle f, A^*\psi_\gamma(x, \cdot)\rangle = \langle Af, \psi_\gamma(x, \cdot)\rangle = \langle g, \psi_\gamma(x, \cdot)\rangle \\ &=: S_\gamma g(x). \end{aligned}$$

The operator S_γ is called the approximate inverse and ψ_γ is the reconstruction kernel. To be precise it is the approximate inverse for approximating the solution f of $Af = g$. If we choose instead of e_γ fulfilling (2.1) a wavelet, then f_γ can be interpreted as a wavelet transform of f. Wavelet transforms are known to approximate in a certain sense derivatives of the transformed function f, see [22]. Hence this is a possibility to find jumps in f as used in contour reconstructions, see [16, 21].

The advantage of this method is that ψ_γ can be pre-computed independently of the data. Furthermore, invariances and symmetries of the operator A^* can be directly transformed into corresponding properties of S_γ as the following consideration shows, see Louis [16]. Let T_1 and T_2 be two operators intertwining with A^*

$$A^*T_2 = T_1A^*.$$

If we choose a standard mollifier E and solve $A^*\Psi = E$ then the solution of Equation (2) for the special mollifier $e_\gamma = T_1 E$ is given as

$$\psi_\gamma = T_2 \Psi.$$

As an example we mention that if A^* is a translation invariant; i.e., $T_1 f(x) = T_2 f(x) = f(x - a)$, then the reconstruction kernel is also a translation invariant.

Sometimes it is easier to cheque these conditions for A itself. Using $AT_1^* = T_2^* A$ we get the above relations by using the adjoint operators.

This method is presented in [17] as a general regularization scheme to solve inverse problems. Generalizations are also given. The application to vector fields is derived by Schuster [31].

If the auxiliary problem is not solvable then its minimum norm solution leads to the minimum norm solution of the original problem.

3 Inversion of the Radon transform

We apply the above approach to derive inversion algorithms for the Radon transform. This represents a typical behaviour for all linear imaging problems. The Radon transform in $\mathbb{R}^N$ is defined as

$$\mathbf{R}f(\theta, s) = \int_{\mathbb{R}^N} f(x)\delta(s - x^\top \theta)\, dx$$

for unit vectors $\theta \in S^{N-1}$ and $s \in \mathbb{R}$. Its inverse is

$$\mathbf{R}^{-1} = c_N \mathbf{R}^* I^{1-N} \tag{3}$$

where $\mathbf{R}^*$ is the adjoint operator from L_2 to L_2, also called the backprojection, defined as

$$\mathbf{R}^* g(x) = \int_{S^{N-1}} g(\theta, x^\top \theta)d\theta,$$

I^α is the Riesz potential defined via the Fourier transform as

$$\widehat{(I^\alpha g)}(\xi) = |\xi|^{-\alpha}\widehat{g}(\xi),$$

acting on the second variable of $\mathbf{R}f$ and the constant

$$c_N = \frac{1}{2}(2\pi)^{1-N},$$

see, e.g., [27]. We start with a mollifier $e_\gamma(x, \cdot)$ for the reconstruction point x and get

$$\mathbf{R}^* \psi_\gamma(x, \cdot) = e_\gamma(x, \cdot)$$
$$= c_N \mathbf{R}^* I^{1-N} \mathbf{R} e_\gamma(x, \cdot)$$

leading to
$$\psi_\gamma(x;\theta,s) = c_N I^{1-N} \mathbf{R}e_\gamma(x;\theta,s).$$

The Radon transform for fixed θ is translational invariant; i.e., if we denote by $\mathbf{R}_\theta f(s) = \mathbf{R}f(\theta,s)$, then
$$\mathbf{R}_\theta T_1^a f = T_2^{a^\top\theta} \mathbf{R}_\theta f$$

with the shift operators $T_1^a f(x) = f(x-a)$ and $T_2^t g(s) = g(s-t)$. If we chose a mollifier $\bar{e}_\gamma$ supported in the unit ball centered around 0 that is shifted to x as
$$e_\gamma(x,y) = 2^{-N} \bar{e}_\gamma(\frac{x-y}{2})$$

then also e_γ is supported in the unit ball and the reconstruction kernel fulfills
$$\psi_\gamma(x;\theta,s) = \frac{1}{2}\bar{\psi}_\gamma(\theta, \frac{s-x^\top\theta}{2})$$

as follows from the general theory in [16] and as was used for the 2D case in [24].

Furthermore, the Radon transform is invariant under rotations; i.e.,
$$\mathbf{R}T_1^U = T_2^U \mathbf{R}$$

for the rotation $T_1^U f(x) = f(Ux)$ with unitary U and $T_2^U g(\theta,s) = g(U\theta,s)$. If the mollifier is invariant under rotation; i.e.,
$$\bar{e}_\gamma(x) = \bar{e}_\gamma(\|x\|)$$

then the reconstruction kernel is independent of θ leading to the following observation.

Theorem 1. *Let the mollifier $e_\gamma(x,y)$ be of the form*
$$e_\gamma(x,y) = 2^{-N}\bar{e}_\gamma(\|x-y\|/2)$$

then the reconstruction kernel is a function only of the variable s and the algorithm is of filtered backprojection type
$$f_\gamma(x) = \int_{S^{n-1}} \int_\mathbb{R} \psi_\gamma(x^\top\theta - s)\mathbf{R}f(\theta,s)ds d\theta. \tag{4}$$

First references to this technique can be found in the work of Grünbaum [2] and Solmon [8].

Lemma 1. *The function f_γ from Theorem 3.1 can be represented as a smoothed inversion or as a reconstruction of smoothed data as*
$$f_\gamma = \mathbf{R}_\gamma^{-1}g = M_\gamma \mathbf{R}^{-1}g = \mathbf{R}^{-1}\tilde{M}g \tag{5}$$

where

$$M_\gamma f(x) = \langle f, e_\gamma(x, \cdot) \rangle$$

and

$$\tilde{M}_\gamma g(\theta, s) = \int_{\mathbb{R}} g(\theta, t) \tilde{e}_\gamma(s - t) dt$$

where

$$\tilde{e}_\gamma(s) = \mathbf{R}e_\gamma(s)$$

for functions e_γ fulfilling the conditions of Theorem 3.1.

4 Optimality criteria

There are several criteria which have to be optimized. The speed of the reconstruction is an essential issue. The scanning time has to be short for the sake of the patients. In order to guarantee a sufficiently high patient throughput, the time for the reconstruction cannot slow down the whole system, but has to be achieved in real-time. The above mentioned invariances adapted to the mathematical model give acceptable results. The speed itself is not sufficient, therefore the accuracy has to be the best possible to ensure the medical diagnosis. This accuracy is determined by the amount of data and of unavoidable noise in the data.

To optimise with respect to accuracy and noise reduction, we consider the problem in suitable Sobolev spaces $H^\alpha = H^\alpha(\mathbb{R}^N)$

$$H^\alpha = \{f \in S' : \|f\|_{H^\alpha}^2 = \int_{\mathbb{R}^N} (1 + |\xi|^2)^\alpha |\hat{f}(\xi)|^2 d\xi < \infty\}.$$

The corresponding norm on the cylinder $C^N = S^{N-1} \times \mathbb{R}$ is evaluated as

$$\|g\|_{H^\alpha(C^N)}^2 = \int_{S^{N-1}} \int_{\mathbb{R}} (1 + |\sigma|^2)^\alpha |\hat{g}(\theta, \sigma)|^2 d\sigma d\theta$$

where the Fourier transform is computed with respect to the second variable. We make the assumption that there is a number $\alpha > 0$ such that

$$c_1 \|f\|_{-\alpha} \leq \|Af\|_{L_2} \leq c_2 \|f\|_{-\alpha}$$

for all $f \in N(A)^\perp$. For the Radon transform in $\mathbb{R}^N$ this holds with $\alpha = (N-1)/2$, see, e.g., [14, 27].

We assume the data to be corrupted by noise; i.e.,

$$g^\varepsilon = \mathbf{R}f + n$$

where the true solution

$$f \in H^\beta$$

and the noise

$$n \in H^t$$

with $t \leq 0$. In the case of white noise, characterized by equal intensity at all frequencies, see, e.g., [10, 15], we hence have $|\hat{n}(\theta, \sigma)| = \text{const}$, and this leads to $n \in H^t$ with $t < -1/2$.

As mollifier we select a low-pass filter in the Fourier domain, resulting in two dimensions in the so-called RAM-LAK-filter. Its disadvantages are described in the next section. The theoretical advantage is that we get information about the frequencies in the solution and therefore the achievable resolution.

This means we select a cut-off $1/\gamma$ for γ sufficiently small and

$$\hat{\tilde{e}}_\gamma(\sigma) = (2\pi)^{-1/2}\chi_{[-1/\gamma, 1/\gamma]}(\sigma)$$

where χ_A denotes the characteristic function of A.

Theorem 2. *Let the true solution be $f \in H^\beta$ with $\|f\|_\beta = \rho$ and the noise be $n \in H^t(C^N)$ with $\|n\|_t = \varepsilon$.*

Then the total error in the reconstruction is for $s < \beta$

$$\|\mathbf{R}_\gamma^{-1}g^\varepsilon - f\|_s \leq c\|n\|_t^{(\beta-s)/(\beta-t+(N-1)/2)}\|f\|_\beta^{(s-t+(N-1)/2)/(\beta-t+(N-1)/2)} \quad (6)$$

when the cut-off frequency is chosen as

$$\gamma = \eta\left(\frac{\|n\|_t}{\|f\|_\beta}\right)^{1/(\beta-t+(N-1)/2)}. \quad (7)$$

Proof. We split the error in the data error and the approximation error as

$$\|\mathbf{R}_\gamma^{-1}g^\varepsilon - f\|_s \leq \|\mathbf{R}_\gamma^{-1}n\|_s + \|\mathbf{R}_\gamma^{-1}\mathbf{R}f - f\|_s.$$

In order to estimate the data error we introduce polar coordinates and apply the so-called projection theorem

$$\hat{f}(\sigma\theta) = (2\pi)^{(1-N)/2}\widehat{\mathbf{R}f}(\theta, \sigma) \quad (8)$$

relating Radon and Fourier transform. With $\widehat{M_\gamma g} = (2\pi)^{1/2}\hat{\tilde{e}}_\gamma\hat{g}$ we get

$$\|\mathbf{R}_\gamma^{-1}n\|_s^2 = (2\pi)^{1-N}\int_{S^{N-1}}\int_{\mathbb{R}}(1+|\sigma|^2)^s\sigma^{N-1}|\widehat{\mathbf{R}\mathbf{R}_\gamma^{-1}n}|^2 d\sigma d\theta$$

$$= (2\pi)^{1-N}\int_{S^{N-1}}\int_{\mathbb{R}}(1+|\sigma|^2)^{s-t}\sigma^{N-1}(1+|\sigma|^2)^t|\widehat{M_\gamma n}|^2 d\sigma d\theta$$

$$\leq (2\pi)^{1-N}\sup_{|\sigma|\leq 1/\gamma}((1+|\sigma|^2)^{s-t}|\sigma|^{N-1})\|n\|_t^2$$

$$= (2\pi)^{1-N}(1+\gamma^{-2})^{s-t}\gamma^{1-N}\|n\|_t^2$$

$$\leq (2\pi)^{1-N}2^{s-t}\gamma^{2(t-s)+1-N}\|n\|_t^2$$

where we have used $\gamma \leq 1$. Starting from $\hat{\tilde{e}}_\gamma = \mathbf{R}e_\gamma$ we compute the Fourier transform of e_γ via the projection theorem as $\hat{e}_\gamma(\xi) = (2\pi)^{-N}\chi_{[0,1/\gamma]}(|\xi|)$ and compute the approximation error as

$$\|\mathbf{R}_\gamma^{-1}\mathbf{R}f - f\|_s = \int_{\mathbb{R}^N} (1 + |\xi|^2)^s |\hat{f}(\xi)|^2 d\xi$$

$$= \int_{|\xi| \geq 1/\gamma} (1 + |\xi|^2)^{(s-\beta)}(1 + |\xi|^2)^\beta |\hat{f}(\xi)|^2 d\xi$$

$$\leq \sup_{|\xi| \geq 1/\gamma} (1 + |\xi|^2)^{(s-\beta)} \|f\|_\beta^2$$

$$\leq \gamma^{2(\beta - s)} \|f\|_\beta^2.$$

The total error is hence estimated as

$$\|\mathbf{R}_\gamma^{-1}g^\varepsilon - f\|_s \leq (2\pi)^{(1-N)/2} 2^{(s-t)/2} \gamma^{(t-s)+(1-N)/2}\|n\|_t + \gamma^{(\beta-s)}\|f\|_\beta.$$

Next we minimize this expression with respect to γ where we put with $a = s - t + (N-1)/2$ and

$$\varphi(\gamma) = c_1 \gamma^{-a}\varepsilon + \gamma^{\beta-s}\rho.$$

Differentiation leads to the minimum at

$$\gamma = \left(\frac{c_1 a\varepsilon}{(\beta - s)\rho}\right)^{1/(\beta-s+a)}.$$

Inserting in φ completes the proof.   □

This result shows that if the data error goes to zero, the cut-off goes to infinity. It is related to the inverse of the signal-to-noise ratio.

5 The filtered backprojection for the Radon transform in 2 and 3 dimensions

In the following we describe the derivation of the filtered backprojection, see Theorem 3.1, for two and three dimensions. As seen in Formula (3.1) the inverse operator of the Radon transform in $\mathbb{R}^N$ has the representation

$$\mathbf{R}^{-1} = \mathbf{R}^* B$$

with

$$B = c_N I^{1-N}.$$

Hence, using

$$e = \mathbf{R}^{-1}\mathbf{R}e = \mathbf{R}^* B\mathbf{R}e = \mathbf{R}^*\psi$$

this can easily be solved as

$$\psi_\gamma = c_N I^{1-N} \mathbf{R} e_\gamma. \tag{9}$$

As mollifier we choose a translational and rotational invariant function

$$\bar{e}_\gamma(x, y) = e_\gamma(\|x - y\|)$$

whose Radon transform then is a function of the variable s only. Taking the Fourier transform of Equation (4.1) we get

$$\hat{\psi}_\gamma(\sigma) = c_N(\widehat{I^{1-N}(\mathbf{R}e_\gamma)})(\sigma)$$
$$= \frac{1}{2}(2\pi)^{(1-N)/2}|\sigma|^{N-1}\hat{e}_\gamma(\sigma),$$

where in the last step we have again used the projection theorem

$$\hat{f}(\sigma\theta) = (2\pi)^{(1-N)/2}\widehat{\mathbf{R}_\theta f}(\sigma).$$

So, we can proceed in the following two ways. Either we prescribe the mollifier e_γ, where the Fourier transform is then computed to

$$\hat{e}_\gamma(\sigma) = \sigma^{1-N/2}\int_0^\infty e_\gamma(s)s^{N/2}J_{N/2-1}(s\sigma)ds$$

where J_ν denotes the Bessel function of order ν. On the other hand we prescribe

$$\hat{e}_\gamma(\sigma) = (2\pi)^{-N/2}F_\gamma(\sigma)$$

with a suitably chosen filter F_γ leading to

$$\hat{\psi}_\gamma(\sigma) = \frac{1}{2}(2\pi)^{1/2-N}|\sigma|^{N-1}F_\gamma(\sigma).$$

If F_γ is the ideal low-pass; i.e., $F_\gamma(\sigma) = 1$ for $|\sigma| \leq \gamma$ and 0 otherwise, then the mollifier is easily computed as

$$e_\gamma(x, y) = (2\pi)^{-N/2}\gamma^N \frac{J_{N/2}(\gamma\|x - y\|)}{(\gamma\|x - y\|)^{N/2}}.$$

In the two-dimensional case, the calculation of ψ leads to the so called RAM-LAK filter, which has the disadvantage of producing ringing artefacts due to the discontinuity in the Fourier domain.

More popular for 2D is the filter

$$F_\gamma(\sigma) = \begin{cases} \text{sinc}\frac{\sigma\pi}{2\gamma}, & |\sigma| \leq \gamma, \\ 0, & |\sigma| > \gamma. \end{cases}$$

From this we compute the kernel ψ_γ by inverse Fourier transform to get $\gamma = \pi/h$ where h is the stepsize on the detector; i.e., $h = 1/q$ if we use $2q + 1$ points on the interval $[-1, 1]$ and $s = s_\ell = \ell h$, $\ell = -q, \ldots, q$

$$\psi_\gamma(s_\ell) = \frac{\gamma^2}{\pi^4} \frac{1}{1 - 4\ell^2},$$

known as Shepp-Logan kernel.

The algorithm of filtered backprojection is a stable discretization of the above described method using the composite trapezoidal rule for computing the discrete convolution. Instead of calculating the convolution for all points $\theta^T x$, the convolution is evaluated for equidistant points ℓh and then a linear interpolation is applied. Nearest neighbour interpolation is not sufficiently accurate, and higher order interpolation is not bringing any improvement because the interpolated functions are not smooth enough. Then the composite trapezoidal rule is used for approximating the backprojection. Here one integrates a periodic function, hence, as shown with the Euler-Maclaurin summation formula, this formula is highly accurate. The filtered backprojection then consists of two steps. Let the data $\mathbf{R}f(\theta, s)$ be given for the directions $\theta_j = (\cos\varphi_j, \sin\varphi_j)$, $\varphi_j = \pi(j-1)/p$, $j = 1, \ldots, p$ and the values $s_k = kh$, $h = 1/q$ and $k = -q, \ldots, q$.

Step 1: For j=1,...,p, evaluate the discrete convolutions

$$v_{j,\ell} = h \sum_{k=-q}^{q} \psi_\gamma(s_\ell - s_k) \mathbf{R}f(\theta_j, s_k), \quad \ell = -q, \ldots, q. \tag{10}$$

Step 2: For each reconstruction point x compute the discrete backprojection

$$\tilde{f}(x) = \frac{2\pi}{p} \sum_{j=1}^{p} ((1 - \eta)v_{j,\ell} + \eta v_{j,\ell+1} \tag{11}$$

where, for each x and j, ℓ and η are determined by

$$s = \theta_j^T x, \ell \le s/h < \ell + 1, \eta = s/h - \ell$$

see, e.g., [27].

In the three-dimensional case we can use the fact, that the operator I^{-2} is local,

$$I^{-2}g(\theta, s) = \frac{\partial^2}{\partial s^2}g(\theta, s).$$

If we want to keep this local structure in the discretization we choose

$$F_\gamma(\sigma) = 2(1 - \cos(h\sigma))/(h\sigma)^2$$

leading to

$$\psi_\gamma(s) = (\delta_\gamma - 2\delta_0 + \delta_{-\gamma})(s). \tag{12}$$

Hence, the application of this reconstruction kernel is nothing but the central difference quotient for approximating the second derivative. The corresponding mollifier then is

$$
e_\gamma(y) = \begin{cases} (2\pi)^{-1}h^{-2}|y|^{-1}, & \text{for } |y| < h, \\ 0, & \text{otherwise,} \end{cases}
$$

see [13]. The algorithm has the same structure as mentioned above for the 2D case.

In order to get reconstruction formulas for the fan beam, geometry coordinate transforms can be used, and the structure of the algorithms does not change.

6 Inversion formula for the 3D cone beam transform

In the following we consider the X-ray reconstruction problem in three dimensions when the data is measured by firing an X-ray tube emitting rays to a 2D detector. The movement of the combination source-detector determines the different scanning geometries. In many real-world applications the source is moved on a circle around the object. From a mathematical point of view this has the disadvantage that the data are incomplete and the condition of Tuy-Kirillov is not fulfilled. This condition says that essentially the data are complete for the three-dimensional Radon transform. More precisely, all planes through a reconstruction point x have to cut the scanning curve Γ. We base our considerations on the assumptions that this condition is fulfilled, the reconstruction from real data is then nevertheless from the above described circular scanning geometry, because other data is not available to us so far.

A first theoretical presentation of the reconstruction kernel was given by Finch [5], and invariances were then used in the group of the author to speed-up the computation time considerably, so that real data could be handled, see [18]. See also the often used algorithm from Feldkamp et al. [4] and the contribution of Defrise and Clack [3]. The approach of Katsevich [9] differs from our approach in that he avoids the Crofton symbol by restricting the back-projection to a range dependent on the reconstruction point x. An overview of the so far existing reconstruction algorithms is given by [34], it is based on a relation between the Fourier transform and the cone beam transform, derived by Tuy [33] generalizing the so-called projection theorem for the Radon transform, see Formula (4.3).

The presentation follows Louis [19].

The mathematical model here is the so-called X-ray transform, where we denote with $a \in \Gamma$ the source position, $\Gamma \subset \mathbb{R}^3$ is a curve, and $\theta \in S^2$ is the direction of the ray:

$$
\mathbf{D}f(a, \theta) = \int_0^\infty f(a + t\theta)\,dt.
$$

The adjoint operator of D as mapping from $L_2(\mathbb{R}^3) \longrightarrow L_2(\Gamma \times S^2)$ is given as

$$\mathbf{D}^*g(x) = \int_\Gamma |x-a|^{-2}g\left(a, \frac{x-a}{|x-a|}\right)da.$$

Most attempts to find inversion formulae are based on a relation between X-ray transform and the 3D Radon transform, the so-called *Formula of Grangeat*, first published in Grangeat's PhD thesis [6], see also [7]:

$$\frac{\partial}{\partial s}\mathbf{R}f(\omega, a^\top\omega) = -\int_{S^2} \mathbf{D}f(a,\theta)\delta'(\theta^\top\omega)d\theta.$$

Proof. We copy the proof from [28]. It consists of the following two steps.
i) We apply the adjoint operator of $\mathbf{R}_\theta$

$$\int_{\mathbb{R}} \mathbf{R}f(\theta, s)\psi(s)ds = \int_{\mathbb{R}^3} f(x)\psi(x^\top\theta)dx.$$

ii) Now we apply the adjoint operator $\mathbf{D}$ for fixed source position a

$$\int_{S^2} \mathbf{D}f(a,\theta)h(\theta)d\theta = \int_{\mathbb{R}^3} f(x)h\left(\frac{x-a}{|x-a|}\right)|x-a|^{-2}dx.$$

Putting in the first formula $\psi(s) = \delta'(s - a^\top\omega)$, using in the second $h(\theta) = \delta'(\theta^\top\omega)$, and the fact that δ' is homogeneous of degree -2 in $\mathbb{R}^3$, then this completes the proof.   □

We note the following rules for δ':
i)

$$\int_{S^2} \psi(a^\top\omega)\delta'(\theta^\top\omega)d\omega = -a^\top\theta \int_{S^2\cap\theta^\perp} \psi'(a^\top\omega)d\omega.$$

ii)

$$\int_{S^2} \psi(\omega)\delta'(\theta^\top\omega)d\omega = -\int_{S^2\cap\theta^\perp} \frac{\partial}{\partial\theta}\psi(\omega)d\omega.$$

Starting point is now the inversion formula for the 3D Radon transform

$$f(x) = -\frac{1}{8\pi^2}\int_{S^2} \frac{\partial^2}{\partial s^2}\mathbf{R}f(\omega, x^\top\omega)d\omega \tag{13}$$

rewritten as

$$f(x) = \frac{1}{8\pi^2}\int_{S^2}\int_{\mathbb{R}} \frac{\partial}{\partial s}\mathbf{R}f(\omega, s)\delta'(s - x^\top\omega)ds d\omega.$$

We assume in the following equation that the Tuy-Kirillov condition is fulfilled. Then we can change the variables as: $s = a^\top\omega$, n is the Crofton symbol; i.e., the number of source points $a \in \Gamma$ such that $a^\top\omega = x^\top\omega$, $m = 1/n$ and get

$$f(x) = \frac{1}{8\pi^2} \int_{S^2} \int_\Gamma (\mathbf{R}f)'(\omega, a^\top \omega)\delta'((a-x)^\top \omega)|a'^\top \omega|m(\omega, a^\top \omega)da d\omega$$

$$= -\frac{1}{8\pi^2} \int_{S^2} \int_\Gamma \int_{S^2} \mathbf{D}f(a,\theta)\delta'(\theta^\top \omega)d\theta\delta'((a-x)^\top \omega)|a'^\top \omega|m(\omega, a^\top \omega)da d\omega$$

$$= -\frac{1}{8\pi^2} \int_\Gamma |x-a|^{-2} \int_{S^2} \int_{S^2} \mathbf{D}f(a,\theta)\delta'(\theta^\top \omega)d\theta\delta'\left(\frac{(x-a)}{|x-a|}^\top \omega\right)$$

$$\times |a'^\top \omega|m(\omega, a^\top \omega)da d\omega$$

where again δ' is homogeneous of degree -2. We now introduce the following operators

$$T_1 g(\omega) = \int_{S^2} g(\theta)\delta'(\theta^\top \omega)d\theta \tag{14}$$

and we use T_1 acting on the second variable as

$$T_{1,a}g(\omega) = T_1 g(a,\omega).$$

We also use the multiplication operator

$$M_{\Gamma,a}h(\omega) = |a'^\top \omega|m(\omega, a^\top \omega)h(\omega), \tag{15}$$

and state the following result.

Theorem 3. *Let the condition of Tuy-Kirillov be fulfilled. Then the inversion formula for the cone beam transform is given as*

$$f = -\frac{1}{8\pi^2}\mathbf{D}^* T_1 M_{\Gamma,a} T_1 \mathbf{D}f \tag{16}$$

with the adjoint operator $\mathbf{D}^*$ of the cone beam transform and T_1 and $M_{\Gamma,a}$ as defined above.

Note that the operators $\mathbf{D}^*$ and M depend on the scanning curve Γ.

This form allows for computing reconstruction kernels. To this end we have to solve the equation

$$D^* \psi_\gamma = e_\gamma$$

in order to write the solution of $\mathbf{D}f = g$ as

$$f(x) = \langle \psi_\gamma(x,\cdot)\rangle.$$

In the case of exact inversion, formula e_γ is the delta distribution. In the case of the approximate inversion formula it is an approximation of this distribution, see the method of approximate inverse. Using $\mathbf{D}^{-1} = -\frac{1}{8\pi^2}\mathbf{D}^* T_1 M_{\Gamma,a} T_1$ we get

$$\mathbf{D}^*\psi = \delta = -\frac{1}{8\pi^2}\mathbf{D}^* T_1 M_{\Gamma,a} T_1 \mathbf{D}\delta$$

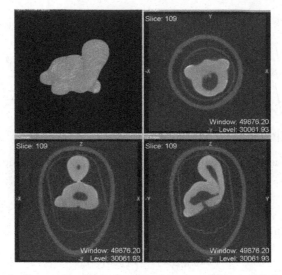

Fig. 1. Reconstruction of a surprise egg with a turtle inside.

and hence

$$\psi = -\frac{1}{8\pi^2}T_1 M_{\Gamma,a}T_1 \mathbf{D}\delta. \tag{17}$$

We can explicitly give the form of the operators T_1 and $T_2 = MT_1$. The index at ∇ indicates the variable with respect to how the differentiation is performed.

$$T_1 g(a,\omega) = \int_{S^2} g(a,\theta)\delta'(\theta^\top \omega)d\theta$$

$$= -\omega^\top \int_{S^2 \cap \omega^\perp} \nabla_2 g(a,\theta)d\theta$$

and

$$T_1 M_{\Gamma,a}h(a,\alpha) = \int_{S^2} \delta'(\omega^\top \alpha)|a'^\top \omega|m(\omega, a^\top \omega)h(a,\omega)d\omega$$

$$= -a'^\top \alpha \int_{S^2 \cap \alpha^\perp} \mathrm{sign}(a'^\top \omega)m(\omega, a^\top \omega)h(a,\omega)d\omega$$

$$-\alpha^\top \int_{S^2 \cap \alpha^\perp} |a'^\top \alpha|\nabla_1 m(\omega, a^\top \omega)h(a,\omega)d\omega$$

$$-a^\top \alpha \int_{S^2 \cap \alpha^\perp} |a'^\top \omega|\nabla_2 m(a, a^\top \omega)h(a,\omega)d\omega$$

$$-\int_{S^2 \cap \alpha^\perp} |a'^\top \omega|m(\omega, a^\top \omega)\frac{\partial}{\partial \alpha}h(a,\omega)d\omega.$$

Note that the function m is piecewise constant and the derivatives are then Delta-distributions at the discontinuities with factor equal to the height of the jump; i.e., $1/2$.

Depending on the scanning curve Γ, invariances have to be used. For the circular scanning geometry this leads to similar results as mentioned in [18]. In Fig. 1 we present a reconstruction from data provided by the Fraunhofer Institut for Nondestructive Testing (IzfP) in Saarbrücken. The detector size was $(204.8mm)^2$ with 512^2 pixels and 400 source positions on a circle around the object. The number of data is 10.4 million. The mollifier used is

$$e_\gamma(y) = (2\pi)^{-3/2}\gamma^{-3}\exp\left(-\frac{1}{2}\left|\frac{y}{\gamma}\right|^2\right).$$

Acknowledgement

The author was supported in part by a Grant of the Hermann und Dr. Charlotte Deutsch Stiftung and by the Deutsche Forschungsgemeinschaft under grant LO 310/8-1.

References

1. A. M. Cormack. Representation of a function by its line integral, with some radiological applications II. *Journal of Applied Physics*, 35:195–207, 1964.
2. M. E. Davison and F. A. Grünbaum. Tomographic reconstruction with arbitrary directions. *IEEE Transactions on Nuclear Science*, 26:77–120, 1981.
3. M. Defrise and R. Clack. A cone-beam reconstruction algorithm using shift-invariant filtering and cone-beam backprojection. *IEEE Transactions on Medical Imaging*, 13:186–195, 1994.
4. L. A. Feldkamp, L. C. Davis, and J. W. Kress. Practical cone beam algorithm. *Journal of the Optical Society of America A*, 6:612–619, 1984.
5. D. Finch. Approximate reconstruction formulae for the cone beam transform, I. Preprint, 1987.
6. P. Grangeat. Analyse d'un système d'imagerie 3D par reconstruction à partir de Radiographics X en géométrie conique. Dissertation, Ecole Nationale Supérieure des Télécommunications, 1987.
7. P. Grangeat. Mathematical framework of cone beam 3-D reconstruction via the first derivative of the radon transform. In G. T. Herman, A. K. Louis, and F. Natterer, editors, *Mathematical Methods in Tomography*, pages 66–97. Springer, Berlin, 1991.
8. I. Hazou and D. C. Solmon. Inversion of the exponential X-ray transform. I: analysis. *Mathematical Methods in the Applied Sciences*, 10:561–574, 1988.
9. A. Katsevich. Analysis of an exact inversion algorithm for spiral-cone beam CT. *Physics in Medicine and Biology*, 47:2583–2597, 2002.
10. H. H. Kuo. *Gaussian measures in Banach spaces*. Number 463 in Lecture Notes in Mathematics. Springer, Berlin, 1975.
11. P. Kuppusamy, M. Chzhan, A. Samouilov, P. Wang, and J. L. Zweier. Mapping the spin-density and lineshape distribution of free radicals using 4D spectral-spatial EPR imaging. *Journal of Magnetic Resonance, Series B*, 197:116–125, 1995.

12. A. K. Louis. Picture reconstruction from projections in restricted range. *Mathematical Methods in the Applied Sciences*, 2:209–220, 1980.
13. A. K. Louis. Approximate inversion of the 3D radon transform. *Mathematical Methods in the Applied Sciences*, 5:176–185, 1983.
14. A. K. Louis. Orthogonal function series expansion and the null space of the Radon transform. *SIAM Journal on Mathematical Analysis*, 15:621–633, 1984.
15. A. K. Louis. *Inverse und schlecht gestellte Probleme*. Teubner, Stuttgart, 1989.
16. A. K. Louis. The approximate inverse for linear and some nonlinear problems. *Inverse Problems*, 12:175–190, 1996.
17. A. K. Louis. A unified approach to regularization methods for linear ill-posed problems. *Inverse Problems*, 15:489–498, 1999.
18. A. K. Louis. Filter design in three-dimensional cone beam tomography: circular scanning geometry. *Inverse Problems*, 19:S31–S40, 2003.
19. A. K. Louis. Development of algorithms in computerized tomography. *AMS Proceedings of Symposia in Applied Mathematics*, 63:25–42, 2006.
20. A. K. Louis and P. Maass. A mollifier method for linear operator equations of the first kind. *Inverse Problems*, 6:427–440, 1990.
21. A. K. Louis and P. Maass. Contour reconstruction in 3D X-ray CT. *IEEE Transactions on Medical Imaging*, TMI12:764–769, 1993.
22. A. K. Louis, P. Maass, and A. Rieder. *Wavelets : Theory and Applications*. Wiley, Chichester, 1997.
23. A. K. Louis and A. Rieder. Incomplete data problems in X-ray computerized tomography, II: Truncated projections and region-of-interest tomography. *Numerische Mathematik*, 56:371–383, 1989.
24. A. K. Louis and T. Schuster. A novel filter design technique in 2D computerized tomography. *Inverse Problems*, 12:685–696, 1996.
25. P. Maass. The X-ray transform: singular value decomposition and resolution. *Inverse Problems*, 3:729–741, 1987.
26. R. B. Marr, C. N. Chen, and P. C. Lauterbur. On two approaches to 3D reconstruction in NMR zeugmatography. In G. T. Herman and F. Natterer, editors, *Mathematical Aspects of Computerized Tomography*, Berlin, 1981. Springer.
27. F. Natterer. *The mathematics of computerized tomography*. Teubner-Wiley, Stuttgart, 1986.
28. F. Natterer and F. Wübbeling. *Mathematical Methods in Image Reconstruction*. SIAM, Philadelphia, 2001.
29. E. T. Quinto. Tomographic reconstruction from incomplete data – numerical inversion of the exterior Radon transform. *Inverse Problems*, 4:867–876, 1988.
30. A. Rieder. Principles of reconstruction filter design in 2d-computerized tomography. *Contemporary Mathematics*, 278:207–226, 2001.
31. T. Schuster. The 3D-Doppler transform: elementary properties and computation of reconstruction kernels. *Inverse Problems*, 16:701–723, 2000.
32. D. Slepian. Prolate spheroidal wave functions, Fourier analysis and uncertainty - V: the discrete case. *Bell System Technical Journal*, 57:1371–1430, 1978.
33. H. K. Tuy. An inversion formula for the cone-beam reconstruction. *SIAM Journal on Applied Mathematics*, 43:546–552, 1983.
34. S. Zhao, H. Yu, and G. Wang. A unified framework for exact cone-beam reconstruction formulas. *Medical Physics*, 32:1712–1721, 2005.

Optimal control in high intensity focused ultrasound surgery

Tomi Huttunen, Jari P. Kaipio, and Matti Malinen

Department of Physics, University of Kuopio, P.O. Box 1627, FIN-70211, Finland
Matti.Malinen@uku.fi

Summary. When an ultrasound wave is focused in biological tissue, a part of the energy of the wave is absorbed and turned into heat. This phenomena is used as a distributed heat source in ultrasound surgery, in which the aim is to destroy cancerous tissue by causing thermal damage. The main advantages of the ultrasound surgery are that it is noninvasive, there are no harmful side effects and spatial accuracy is good. The main disadvantage is that the treatment time is long for large cancer volumes when current treatment techniques are used. This is due to the undesired temperature rise in healthy tissue during the treatment. The interest for optimization of ultrasound surgery has been increased recently. With proper mathematical models and optimization algorithms the treatment time can be shortened and temperature rise in tissues can be better localized. In this study, two alternative control procedures for thermal dose optimization during ultrasound surgery are presented. In the first method, the scanning path between individual foci is optimized in order to decrease the treatment time. This method uses the prefocused ultrasound fields and predetermined focus locations. In the second method, combined feedforward and feedback controls are used to produce desired thermal dose in tissue. In the feedforward part, the phase and amplitude of the ultrasound transducers are changed as a function of time to produce the desired thermal dose distribution in tissue. The foci locations do not need to be predetermined. In addition, inequality constraint approximations for maximum input amplitude and maximum temperature can be used with the proposed method. The feedforward control is further expanded with a feedback controller which can be used during the treatment to compensate the modeling errors. All of the proposed control methods are tested with numerical simulations in 2D or 3D.

Keywords: Ultrasound surgery, optimal control, minimum time control, feedforward control, feedback control.

1 Introduction

In high intensity focused ultrasound surgery (HIFU), the cancerous tissue in the focal region is heated up to 50–90°C. Due to the high temperature, thermal dose in tissue raises in a few seconds to the level that causes necrosis [43, 44].

Furthermore, the effect of the diffusion and perfusion can be minimized with high temperature and short sonication time [26]. In the current procedure of ultrasound surgery, the tissue is destroyed by scanning the cancerous volume point by point using predetermined individual foci [14]. The position of the focus is changed either by moving the transducer mechanically, or by changing the phase and amplitude of individual transducer elements when a phased array is used. The thermal information during the treatment is obtained via magnetic resonance imaging (MRI) [7]. This procedure is efficient for the treatment of small tumor volumes. However, as the tumor size increases and treatment is accomplished by temporal switching between foci, the temperature in healthy tissue accumulates and can cause undesired damage [9, 17]. This problem has increased the interest toward the detailed optimization of the treatment. With control and optimization methods, it is possible to decrease the treatment time as well as to control the temperature or thermal dose in both healthy and cancerous tissue.

The different approaches have been proposed to control and optimize temperature or thermal dose in ultrasound surgery. For temperature control, a linear quadratic regulator (LQR) feedback controller was proposed in [21]. In that study, controller parameters were adjusted as a function of time according to absorption in focus. The controller was designed to keep temperature in focus point at a desired level. Another LQR controller was proposed in [46]. That controller was also designed to keep the temperature in single focus point at a predetermined level, and the tissue parameters for the controller were estimated with MRI temperature data before the actual treatment.

The direct control of the thermal dose gives several advantages during ultrasound surgery. These advantages are reduced peak temperature, decreased applied power and decreased overall treatment time [13]. The proposed thermal dose optimization approaches include power adjusted focus scans [47], weighting approach [22] and temporal switching between single [17] or multiple focus patterns [13]. In all of these studies, only a few predetermined focus patterns were used, i.e., thermal dose was optimized by choosing the treatment strategy from the small set of possible paths or focus distributions. Finally, model predictive control (MPC) approach for thermal dose optimization was proposed in [1]. In the MPC approach, the difference between the desired thermal dose and current thermal dose was weighted with a quadratic penalty. Furthermore, the modeling errors in perfusion can be decreased with MRI temperature data during the control. However, the MPC approach was proposed for the predetermined focus points and scanning path, and it is computationally expensive, especially in 2D and 3D.

In this study, alternative methods for optimization and control of the thermal dose are presented. The first method concerns scanning path optimization between individual foci. In this approach, the cancer volume is filled with a predetermined set of focal points, and focused ultrasound fields are computed for each focus. The optimization algorithm is then constructed as the minimum time formulation of the optimal control theory [20, 42]. The proposed algorithm optimizes the scanning path, i.e., finds the order in which foci are treated. The proposed optimization method uses the linear state equation and it is computationally easy to implement to current clinical machinery. The scanning path optimization method can be also used with MRI temperature feedback. The details of this method can be found from [34]. The simulations from the optimized scanning path show that treatment time can be efficiently decreased as compared to the current scanning technique. In the current technique, the treatment is usually started from the outermost focus and foci are scanned by the decreasing order of the distance between the outermost focus and transducer.

The second method investigated here is a combination of model based feedforward control and feedback control to compensate modeling errors. In feedforward control the thermal dose distribution in tissue is directly optimized by changing the phase and amplitude of the ultrasound transducers as a function of time. The quadratic penalty is used to weight the difference between the current thermal dose and desired thermal dose. The inequality constraint approximations for the maximum input amplitude and maximum temperature are included in the design. This approach leads to a large dimension nonlinear control problem which is solved using gradient search [42]. The proposed feedforward control method has several advantages over other optimization procedures. First, the thermal dose can be optimized in both healthy and cancerous tissue. Second, the variation of diffusion and perfusion values in different tissues is taken into account. Third, the latent thermal dose which accumulates after the transducers have been turned off can be taken into account. The feedforward control method is discussed in detail in [32] for temperature control and in [33] for thermal dose optimization. In the second part of the overall control procedure, a linear quadratic Gaussian (LQG) controller with Kalman filter for state estimation is used to compensate the modeling errors which may appear in the feedforward control. The temperature data for the feedback can be adopted from MRI during the treatment. The feedback controller is derived by linearizing the original nonlinear control problem with respect to the feedforward trajectories for temperature and control input. The LQG controller and Kalman filter are then derived from these linearized equations. The details of the LQG feedback control can be found in [31].

In this study, numerical examples for each control procedure are presented. All examples concern the ultrasound surgery of breast cancer, and the modeling is done either in 2D or 3D. The potential of ultrasound surgery for the treatment of breast cancer is shown in clinical studies in [18] and [27]. Although all examples concern the ultrasound surgery of the breast, there are no limitations to using derived methods in the ultrasound surgery of other organs, see for example [33].

2 Mathematical models

2.1 Wave field model

The first task in the modeling of ultrasound surgery is to compute the ultrasound field. If acoustic parameters of tissue are assumed to be homogeneous, the time harmonic ultrasound field can be computed from the Rayleigh integral [39]. If the assumption of the homogeneity is not valid, the pressure field can be obtained as a solution of the Helmholtz equation. The Helmholtz equation in inhomogeneous absorbing media can be written as

$$\nabla \cdot \left(\frac{1}{\rho}\nabla p\right) + \frac{\kappa^2}{\rho}p = 0, \tag{1}$$

where ρ is density, c is the speed of sound and $\kappa = 2\pi f/c + i\alpha$, where f is the frequency and α is the absorption coefficient [4].

The Helmholtz equation with suitable boundary conditions can be solved with a variety of methods. Traditional approaches include the low-order finite element method (FEM) and the finite difference method (FD) [28]. The main limitation of these methods is that they require several elements per wavelength to obtain a reliable solution. At high frequency ultrasound computations, this requirement leads to very large dimensional numerical problems. To avoid this problem ray approximations have been used to compute ultrasound field [5, 16, 29]. However, the complexity of ray approximation increases dramatically in complex geometries in the presence of multiple material interfaces.

An alternative approach for ultrasound wave modeling is to use the improved full wave methods, such as the pseudo-spectral [48] and k-space methods [35]. In addition, there are methods in which a priori information of the approximation subspace can be used. In the case of the Helmholtz equation, a priori information is usually plane wave basis which is a solution of the homogeneous Helmholtz equation. The methods which use plane wave basis include the partition of unity method (PUM) [2], least squares method [37], wave based method (Trefftz method) [45] and ultra weak variational formulation (UWVF) [6, 24].

In this study, the Helmholtz equation (1) is solved using the UWVF. The computational issues of UWVF are discussed in detail in [24], and UWVF approximation is used in the related ultrasound surgery control problems in [32] and [33]. The main idea in UWVF is to use plane wave basis functions from different directions in the elements of standard FEM mesh. The variational form is formulated in the element boundaries, thus reducing integration task in assembling the system matrices. Finally, the resulting UWVF matrices have a sparse block structure. These properties make the UWVF a potential solver for high frequency wave problems.

2.2 Thermal evolution model

The temperature in biological tissues can be modeled with the Pennes bioheat equation [38]

$$\rho C_T \frac{\partial T}{\partial t} = \nabla \cdot k\nabla T - w_B C_B(T - T_A) + Q, \tag{2}$$

where $T = T(r,t)$ is the temperature in which $r = r(x,y,z)$ is the spatial variable. Furthermore, in Equation (2) C_T is the heat capacity of tissue, k is the diffusion coefficient, w_B is the arterial perfusion, C_B is the heat capacity of blood, T_A is the arterial blood temperature and Q is the heat source term. The heat source for time-harmonic acoustic pressure can be defined as [39]

$$Q = \alpha \frac{|p|^2}{\rho c}. \tag{3}$$

If the wave fields for the heat source are computed from the Helmholtz equation, the heat source term can be written as

$$Q = \frac{\alpha(r)}{\rho(r)c(r)}|p(r,t)|^2 = \frac{\alpha(r)}{\rho(r)c(r)}\left|\sum_{k=1}^{m} \tilde{u}_k(t)\tilde{C}_k(r)\right|^2, \tag{4}$$

where $\tilde{u}_k(t) \in \mathbb{C}$ determines the amplitude and phase of the transducer number k and $\tilde{C}_k(r) \in \mathbb{C}^N$ is the time-harmonic solution of the Helmholtz problem, where N is the number of spatial discretization points.

The bioheat equation can be solved using the standard FEM [12, 36] or FD-time domain methods [8, 11]. In this study, the semi-discrete FEM with the implicit Euler time integration is used to solve the bioheat equation. The detailed FEM formulation of the bioheat equation can be found in [32] and [33]. The implicit Euler form of the bioheat equation can be written as

$$T_{t+1} = AT_t + P + M_D(Bu_t)^2, \tag{5}$$

where $T_t \in \mathbb{R}^N$ is the FEM approximation of temperature, matrix $A \in \mathbb{R}^{N \times N}$ arises from the discretization of FEM and vector P is related to perfusion term. The heat source term $M_D(Bu_t)^2 \in \mathbb{R}^N$ is constructed from the precomputed ultrasound fields as follows. The real and imaginary parts of the variable $\tilde{u}_k(t)$ in Equation (4) are separated as $u_k = \mathrm{Re}\,\tilde{u}_k$ and $u_{m+k} = \mathrm{Im}\,\tilde{u}_k$, $k = 1, ..., m$, resulting in the control variable vector $u(t) \in \mathbb{R}^{2m}$. Furthermore, solutions of the Helmholtz problem are arranged as $\hat{C}_k = (\tilde{C}_k(r_1), ..., \tilde{C}_k(r_N))^T$ and $\hat{C} = (\hat{C}_1, ..., \hat{C}_m) \in \mathbb{C}^{N \times m}$. For control purposes, the matrix $\hat{C}$ is written in the form where real and imaginary parts of the wave fields are separated as

$$B = \begin{pmatrix} \mathrm{Re}\,\hat{C} & -\mathrm{Im}\,\hat{C} \\ \mathrm{Im}\,\hat{C} & \mathrm{Re}\,\hat{C} \end{pmatrix} \in \mathbb{R}^{2N \times 2m}. \tag{6}$$

In Equation (5), matrix $M_D \in \mathbb{R}^{N \times 2m}$ is the modified mass matrix which is constructed as $M_D = [I, I]M$, where I is the unit matrix. In addition, the square of the heat source term in Equation (5) is computed element wisely. With this procedure, it is possible to control the real and imaginary parts (phase and amplitude) of each transducer element separately. For detailed derivation of the heat source term, see example [33].

In this study, the boundary condition for the FE bioheat equation (5) was chosen as the Dirichlet condition in all simulations. In the Dirichlet condition, the temperature on the boundaries of the computational domain was set to 37°C. Furthermore, the initial condition for the implicit Euler iteration was set as $T_0 = 37$°C in all simulated cases.

2.3 Thermal dose model

The combined effect of the temperature and the treatment time can be evaluated using the thermal dose. For biological tissues thermal dose is defined as [40]

$$D(T(r, \cdot)) = \int_0^{t_f} R^{\left(43 - T(r,t)\right)} \, dt\,, \quad \text{where } R = \begin{cases} 0.25 & \text{for } T(r,t) < 43°\text{C} \\ 0.50 & \text{for } T(r,t) \geq 43°\text{C} \end{cases} \tag{7}$$

and t_f is the final time where thermal dose is integrated. The unit of the thermal dose is equivalent minutes at 43°C. In most of the soft tissues the thermal dose that causes thermal damage is between 50 and 240 equivalent minutes at 43°C [10, 11].

3 Control and optimization algorithms for ultrasound surgery

In the following, different control and optimization algorithms for thermal dose and temperature control in ultrasound surgery are presented. The numerical simulations are given after the theoretical part of each algorithm.

3.1 Scanning path optimization method

In the scanning path optimization algorithm, the heat source term in the implicit Euler FEM form of the bioheat equation (5) is linearized. In this case, a new matrix $\widetilde{B} \in \mathbb{R}^{N \times N_f}$ is constructed from focused ultrasound fields, where the number of foci is N_f. The mass matrix M is also included to matrix the $\widetilde{B}$. With these changes, the bioheat equation is written as

$$T_{t+1} = AT_t + P + \widetilde{B}_t u_t, \tag{8}$$

where $\widetilde{B}_t \in \mathbb{R}^N$ is the active field at time t and u_t is the input power. The active field $(\widetilde{B}_t)$ at time t is taken as a column from the matrix $\widetilde{B}$ in which focused fields for predetermined foci are set as columns. The cost function for the scanning path optimization can be set as a terminal condition

$$J(D) = (D - D_d)^T W (D - D_d), \tag{9}$$

where the difference between thermal dose and desired thermal dose D_d is penalized using positive definite matrix W. The Hamiltonian form for the state equation (8) and the cost function (9) can be written as [38]

$$H(D, T, u) = \|D - D_d\|_W^2 + \lambda_t^T (AT_t - P + \widetilde{B}u_t), \tag{10}$$

where $\lambda_t \in \mathbb{R}^N$ is the Lagrange multiplier for the state equation. The optimization problem can be solved from the costate equation [42]

$$\lambda_{t-1} = \frac{\partial H}{\partial T_t} = A^T \lambda_t + \log(R) R^{43 - T_t} \odot W (D - D_d), \tag{11}$$

where $\odot$ is the element wise (Hadamard) product of two vectors. The costate equation is computed backwards in time. The focus which minimizes the cost function (9) at time t can be found as

$$\min\{\lambda_t^T \widetilde{B}\}, \tag{12}$$

so the focus which is chosen makes Equation (12) most negative at time t [20, 42]. The feedback law can be chosen as maximum effort feedback

$$u_{t+1} = \begin{cases} T_d - T_{i,t}, & \text{if } \lambda_t^T \widetilde{B} < 0, \\ 0, & \text{if } \lambda_t^T \widetilde{B} \geq 0, \end{cases} \tag{13}$$

where $T_{i,t}$ is temperature at i^{th} focus point at time t, and T_d is the desired temperature in the cancer region. In this study, the desired temperature in the cancer region was set to $T_d = 70°C$.

The scanning path optimization algorithm consists of the following steps: 1) Solve the state equation (8) from time t upwards in a predetermined time window. 2) Solve the Lagrange multiplier from Equation (11) backwards in the same time window. 3) Find the next focus point from Equation (12). 4) Compute the input value from Equation (13). If the target is not fully treated, return to step 1).

3.2 Scanning path optimization simulations

The scanning path optimization method was evaluated in two schematic 3D geometries, which are shown in Figure 1. In both geometries, the ultrasound surgery of the breast was simulated. In the first geometry, there are skin,

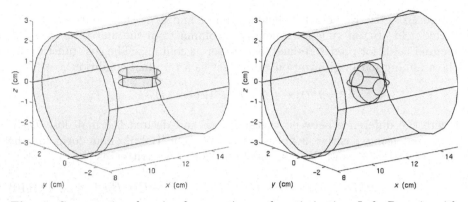

Fig. 1. Computation domains for scanning path optimization. Left: Domain with the slice target. Right: Domain with the sphere target. The subdomains from left to right are skin, healthy breast and cancer.

Table 1. Thermal parameters for subdomains.

Subdomain	α(Nep/m)	k(W/mK)	C_T(J/kgK)	w_B(kg/m³s)
skin	30	0.5	3770	1
breast	5	0.5	3550	0.5
cancer	5	0.5	3770	10

healthy breast and slice shaped target, with the radius of 1 cm. In the second geometry, the subdomains are the same, but the target is a sphere with the radius of 1 cm. Both targets were located so that the center of the target was at the point (12,0,0) cm. The computation domains were partitioned into the following meshes. With the slice target, the mesh consists of 13,283 vertices and the 70,377 elements and with the spherical target the mesh consists of 24,650 vertices and 13,4874 elements.

The transducer system in simulations was a 530-element phased array (Figure 2). The transducer was located so that the center of the target was in the geometrical focus. The ultrasound fields with the frequency of 1 MHz were computed for each element using the Rayleigh integral. The acoustical properties of tissue were set as c=1500 m/s, ρ=1000 kg/m³ and α=5 Nep/m [15, 19]. The thermal properties of tissue are given in Table 1, and these properties were also adopted from the literature [25, 30, 41].

In the control problem, the objective was to obtain the thermal dose of 300 equivalent minutes at 43°C in the whole target domain and keep the thermal dose in healthy regions as low as possible. A transition zone with the thickness of 0.5 cm was used around the target volume. In this region, the thermal dose was not limited. The maximum temperature in healthy tissue was limited to 44°C. If this temperature was reached, the tissue was allowed to cool to 42.5°C or below.

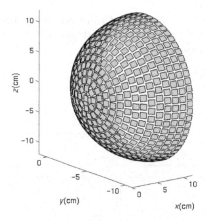

Fig. 2. 530-element phased array used in simulations.

The weighting matrix W for the thermal dose difference was set to a diagonal matrix. The weights on the diagonal were set adaptively in the following way. The total number of foci was denoted with N_f and the number of foci in which the desired thermal dose was reached was denoted with N_d. The vertices in healthy subdomains were weighted with the function $10,000 \times (1 - N_d/N_f)^2$, and the vertices in the cancerous domain with $(1 - N_d/N_f)^{-2}$, i.e., the weighting from the healthy region was decreased and correspondingly increased in the target during the treatment. In addition, when the thermal dose of 300 equivalent minutes was reached, the weighting from this focus was removed. The implicit Euler form of the bioheat equation (8) was adopted by setting the time step as $h=0.25$ s for the slice target and $h=0.5$ s for the sphere target. The scanning path was chosen using the algorithm described in the previous section. The time window for state and costate equations were chosen to be 10 s upwards from the current time.

Simulated results were compared to the treatment where scanning is started from the outermost focus (in x-coordinate) and the target volume is then scanned in decreasing order of the x-coordinate. For example, in the 3D case, the outermost untreated location in the x-coordinate was chosen and then the corresponding slice in y- and z-directions was sonicated. The feedback law and temperature constraints were the same for the optimized scanning path and this reference method. Furthermore, if the dose at the next focus location was above the desired level, this focus was skipped (i.e., power was not wasted). In the following, the results from this kind of sonication are referred to as "standard sonication." For both of the methods, the treatment was terminated when the thermal dose of 300 equivalent minutes was reached in the whole target.

The foci in target volumes were chosen so that the minimum distance in each direction from focus to focus was 1 mm. For the slice target, the foci were located in $z=0$ plane, while with the spherical target, the whole volume was covered with foci.

Table 2. Results from the scanning path optimization. The number of the foci in target is N_f and t is the treatment time. Subscript O refers to optimized scanning path and S to standard sonication.

Case	N_f	t_O (s)	t_S (s)
Slice	158	41	58
Sphere	816	493	866

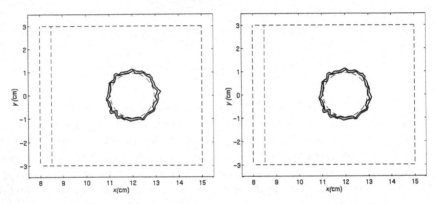

Fig. 3. Thermal dose contours for the slice scan in xy-plane. Left: Thermal dose contours with optimized scanning path. Right: Thermal dose contours with standard sonication. The contour lines are for 240 and 120 equivalent minutes at $43°$ C.

The treatment times for the optimized scanning path and standard sonication are given in Table 2. The sonication time is 30% shorter for the slice target and 44% shorter for the sphere shaped target as compared to standard sonication. The treatment time is reduced more for the spherical target, since the degrees of freedom for the optimization algorithm are increased in 3D.

The thermal dose contours in xy-plane for the slice shaped target are shown in Figure 3. With both of the methods, the desired thermal dose is achieved well into the target region. In addition, the thermal dose decreases efficiently in the transition zone and there are no undesired thermal doses in healthy regions.

The maximum temperature trajectories for the target and healthy domains for the slice target are shown in Figure 4. This figure shows that the whole target volume can be treated using a single sonication burst with both of the methods. With scanning path optimization, the maximum temperature in healthy domains is smaller than with the standard sonication.

The thermal dose contours for the spherical target in different planes are shown in Figure 5. Again, the therapeutically relevant thermal dose is achieved in the whole target volume, and there are no big differences in dose contours between optimized and standard scanning methods.

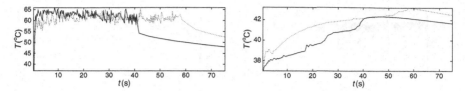

Fig. 4. Maximum temperatures for the slice scan. Left: Maximum temperature in cancer. Right: Maximum temperature in healthy tissue. Solid line is for optimized scan and dotted for standard sonication.

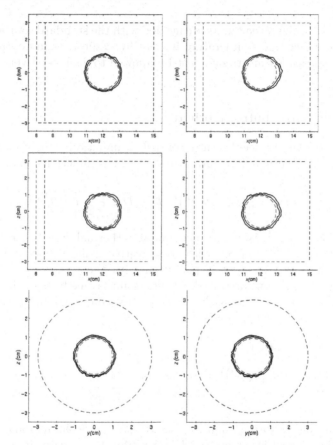

Fig. 5. Thermal dose contours for the spherical scan in different planes. Left column: Thermal dose contours from optimized scanning path. Right column: Thermal dose contours from the standard sonication. The contour lines are for 240 and 120 equivalent minutes at $43°C$.

The maximum temperature trajectories for the target and healthy tissue from the spherical scan are shown in Figure 6. This figure indicates that the treatment can be accomplished much faster by using the optimized scanning path. The optimized scanning path needs three sonication bursts to treat the

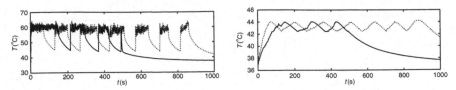

Fig. 6. Maximum temperatures for the sphere scan. Left: Maximum temperature in cancer. Right: Maximum temperature in healthy tissue. Solid line is for optimized scan and dotted for standard sonication.

whole cancer, while seven bursts are needed with the standard sonication. This is due to the fact that temperature in healthy tissue rises more rapidly with standard sonication, and tissue must be allowed to cool to prevent undesired damage.

3.3 Feedforward control method

The first task in the feedforward control formulation is to define the cost function. In the thermal dose optimization, the cost function can be written as

$$J(D, \dot{u}; t) = \frac{1}{2}(D - D_d)^T W (D - D_d) + \frac{1}{2}\int_0^{t_f} \dot{u}_t^T S \dot{u}_t \, dt, \qquad (14)$$

where the difference between the accumulated thermal dose D and the desired thermal dose D_d is weighted with the positive definite matrix W and the time derivative of the input is penalized with the positive definite matrix S. The maximum input amplitude of ultrasound transducers is limited. This limitation can be handled with an inequality constraint approximation, in which k^{th} component $c_{1,k}(u_t)$ is

$$c_{1,k}(u_t) = c_{1,m+k}(u_t) \qquad (15)$$
$$= \begin{cases} K\left(\left(u_{k,t}^2 + u_{m+k,t}^2(t)\right)^{1/2} - u_{\max,i}\right)^2, & \text{if } \left(u_{k,t}^2 + u_{m+k,t}^2\right)^{1/2} \geq u_{\max,i}, \\ 0, & \text{if}\left(u_{k,t}^2 + u_{m+k,t}^2\right)^{1/2} < u_{\max,i}, \end{cases}$$

where K is the weighting scalar, $u_{k,t}$ and $u_{m+k,t}$ are the real and imaginary parts of the control input for the kth transducer, respectively, $u_{\max,i}$ is the maximum amplitude during the ith interval of the sonication and $k = 1, \ldots, m$. With this manner it is possible to split treatment into several parts when transducers are alternatively on or off. For example, when large cancer volumes are treated, the healthy tissue can be allowed to cool between the sonication bursts. Furthermore, in feedforward control, it is useful to set the maximum amplitude limitation lower than what transducers can actually produce. With this manner it is possible to leave some reserve power for feedback purposes to compensate for the modeling errors.

In practice, there are also limitations for the maximum temperature in both healthy and cancerous tissue. The pain threshold is reported to be approximately 45°C. In addition, the temperature in cancerous tissue must be below the water boiling temperature (100°C). These limitations can be made in the form of an inequality constraint approximation c_2, whose i^{th} component is

$$c_{2,i}(T_t) = \begin{cases} K(T_{i,t} - T_{\max,C})^2, & \text{if } T_{i,t} \in \Omega_C \quad \text{and } T_{i,t} \geq T_{\max,\Omega_C}, \\ K(T_{i,t} - T_{\max,H})^2, & \text{if } T_{i,t} \in \Omega_H \quad \text{and } T_{i,t} \geq T_{\max,\Omega_H}, \\ 0, & \text{otherwise.} \end{cases} \quad (16)$$

where T_i is the temperature in the FE vertex i, the subset of the vertices in cancerous region is denoted by Ω_C and the subset of the vertices in the healthy region is denoted by Ω_H. The maximum allowed temperature is denoted in cancerous and healthy tissue by $T_{\max,\Omega_C}$ and $T_{\max,\Omega_H}$, respectively.

The feedforward control problem solution can be obtained via the Hamiltonian form [42]. Combining equations (14), (5), (15) and (16) gives the Hamiltonian

$$H(T, u, \dot{u}; t) = \frac{1}{2}\left((D - D_d)^T W(D - D_d) + \int_0^{t_f} \dot{u}_t^T S\dot{u}_t dt\right)$$
$$+ \lambda_t^T\left(AT_t - P - M_D(Bu_t)^2\right) + \mu_t^T c_1(u_t) + \nu_t^T c_2(T_t), \quad (17)$$

where μ_t is the Lagrange multiplier for the control input inequality constraint approximation and ν_t is the Lagrange multiplier for the temperature inequality constraint approximation.

The feedforward control problem can be now solved by using a gradient search algorithm. This algorithm consists of following steps: 1) Compute the state equation (5). 2) Compute the Lagrange multiplier for the state as $-\lambda_t = \partial H / \partial T_t$ backwards in time. 3) Compute the Lagrange multiplier for the control input inequality constraint as $\mu_t = (\partial c_1/\partial u_t)^{-1}(\partial H/\partial u_t)$. 4) Compute the Lagrange multiplier for the temperature inequality constraint using the penalty function method as $\nu_t = \partial c_2/\partial T_t$. 5) Compute the stationary condition. For the ℓth iteration round, the stationary condition (input update) can be computed as $u_t^{(\ell+1)} = u_t^{(\ell)} + \epsilon^{(\ell)} \partial H/\partial u_t^{(\ell)}$, where $\epsilon^{(\ell)}$ is the iteration step length. 6) Compute the value of the cost function from Equation (14). If the change in the cost function is below a predetermined value, stop iteration, otherwise return to step 1.

3.4 Feedforward control simulations

2D example

The computational domain in this example was chosen as a part of a cancerous breast, see Figure 7. The domain was divided into four subdomains which are

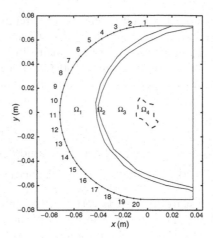

Fig. 7. Computational domain. Cancerous region is marked with the dashed line (Ω_4). Twenty ultrasound transducers are numbered on the left hand side.

Table 3. The acoustic and thermal parameters for the feedforward control simulation.

Domain	α (Nep/m)	c (m/s)	ρ (kg/m³s)	k (W/mK)	C_T (J/kgK)	w_B (kg/m³s)
Ω_1	0	1500	1000	0.60	4190	0
Ω_2	12	1610	1200	0.50	3770	1
Ω_3	5	1485	1020	0.50	3550	0.7
Ω_4	5	1547	1050	0.65	3770	2.3

water (Ω_1), skin (Ω_2) a part of a healthy breast (Ω_3) and the breast tumor (Ω_4). The domain was partitioned into a mesh having 2108 vertices and 4067 elements.

The transducers system was chosen as a 20-element phased array (see Figure 7). The transducer was located so that the center of the cancer was in the geometrical focus. The frequency of ultrasound fields was set to 500 kHz. The wave fields were computed using the UWVF for each transducer element. The acoustic and thermal parameters for the subdomains were adopted from the literature [3, 30, 41] and they are given in Table 3. It is worth noting that the frequency in this example was chosen lower than in scanning path optimization simulations, and the absorption coefficient in skin is therefore lower.

The feedforward control objective was to obtain the thermal dose of 300 equivalent minutes at 43°C in the cancer region and below 120 equivalent minutes in healthy regions. The transient zone near the cancer, where thermal dose is allowed to rise, was not included to this simulation. The reason for this is the testing of the spatial accuracy of controller. The weighting for thermal dose distribution was chosen as follows. The weighting matrix W was set to diagonal matrix and the nodes in the skin, healthy breast and cancer were weighted with 500, 2500 and 2000, respectively.

For feedforward control problem, the time interval $t=[0,180]$ s was discretized with the step length $h=0.5$ s and the treatment was split into two parts. During the first part of the sonication (i.e., when $t \in [0,50]$ s) the maximum amplitude was limited with $u_{max,1}=0.8$ MPa, and during the second part (i.e., when $t \in [50,180]$ s) the maximum amplitude was limited with $u_{max,2}=0.02$ MPa. In the inequality constraint approximation for maximum amplitude, the weighting was set to $K=10,000$. The smoothing of the transducer excitations was achieved by setting the weighting matrix for time derivative of the control input as $S=\mathrm{diag}(5000)$. In this simulation, the maximum temperature inequality constraint approximation was not used, i.e., $c_{2,t} = 0$ for all t. The thermal dose was optimized using the algorithm described in previous section. The iteration was stopped when the relative change in cost function was below 10^{-4}.

The thermal dose contours for the region of interest are shown in Figure 8. These contours indicate that the major part of the thermal dose is in the cancer area and only a small fraction of the dose is in the healthy breast. The thermal dose of 240 equivalent minutes at 43°C is achieved in 74% of the target area and 120 equivalent minutes at 92% of the cancer area. In the breast, only 2.4% of the area has thermal dose of 120 equivalent minutes. The maximum thermal dose peak in the breast is quite high. However, this dose peak is found only in a small part of the breast. In this simulation the modeling of cooling period between [50 180] s is crucial, since 75% of the thermal dose is accumulated during this time.

The phase and amplitude trajectories for the transducers number 4 and 16 are shown in Figure 9. There are no oscillations in the phase and amplitude trajectories, so design criterion concerning this limitation is fulfilled.

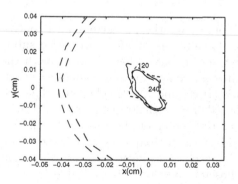

Fig. 8. The feedforward controlled dose at the final time ($t_f=180$ s). Contour lines are for 120 and 240 equivalent minutes at 43°C.

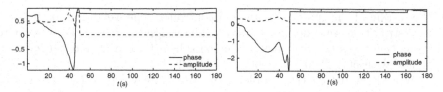

Fig. 9. Phase and amplitude trajectories from the feedforward control for transducer number 4 (left) and 16 (right).

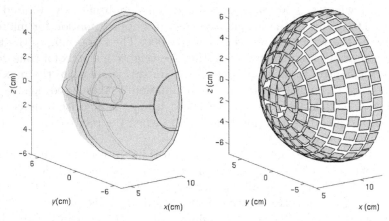

Fig. 10. Left: Computation domain. Subdomains from the left are skin, healthy breast and the sphere shaped cancer. Right: 200-element phased array.

Furthermore, the maximum input amplitude during the first part of sonication was 0.801 MPa and during the second part 0.0203 MPa, so the maximum amplitude inequality constraint approximation limits the amplitude with a tolerable accuracy.

3D example

The computation domain for the 3D feedforward control problem is shown in Figure 10. The domain was divided into three subdomains which were skin, healthy breast and a sphere shaped cancer with the radius of 1 cm at the point (7,0,0) cm. The computational domain was partitioned into a mesh consisting of 23,716 vertices and 120,223 elements. The transducer system was a hemispherical phased array with 200 elements (see Figure 7). The transducer was located so that the center of the target was in the geometrical focus. The ultrasound fields with the frequency of 1 MHz were computed using the Rayleigh integral for each transducer element. The acoustical and thermal parameters were chosen as Section 3.2 (see Table 1).

The control problem was to obtain the thermal dose of 300 equivalent minutes or greater at 43°C in the cancer region. The temperature in the healthy tissue was limited to 45°C and to 80°C in cancer, with the inequality constraint approximation. In this simulation, a 0.5 cm transient zone was set between the cancer and healthy tissue, where temperature or thermal dose was not limited, since temperature in the simulation in this region was less than 80°C. The weighting matrix W was set to diagonal matrix, and the vertices in cancer region were weighted with 10,000 and other nodes had zero weights.

For the feedforward control problem, the time interval $t=[0,50]$ s was discretized with step length $h=0.5$ s and the treatment was split to two parts. During the first part of the sonication (i.e., when $t \in [0,30]$ s), the maximum amplitude was limited with $u_{max,1}=100$ kPa and during the second part (i.e., when $t \in [30,50]$ s), the maximum amplitude was limited with $u_{max,2}=2$ kPa. The diagonal weighting matrix S for the time derivative of the input was set to $S=\text{diag}(10,000)$. The weighting scalar for both state and input inequality constraint approximations was set to $K = 2 \times 10^6$. The stopping criterion for feedforward control iteration was that the thermal dose of 240 equivalent minutes was achieved in the whole cancer.

The thermal dose contours from the feedforward control are shown in Figure 11. As it can be seen, the thermal dose of 240 equivalent minutes is achieved in the whole cancer region. Furthermore, the thermal dose is sharply localized in the cancer region. There are no undesired doses in the healthy regions. In this simulation, the thermal dose accumulation during the cooling period ($t \in [30, 50]$) was 11% of the whole thermal dose.

The temperature trajectories for cancer and healthy tissue are shown in Figure 12. From this figure it can be seen that the temperature in cancer regions is limited to 80°C. Also, the maximum temperature in healthy regions is near 45°C. The maximum temperature in the cancer was 80.3°C and in the healthy region 45.5°C. Furthermore, the maximum input amplitude inequality constraint approximation was found to be effective. The maximum amplitude during the first part of the sonication was 101 kPa and 2.02 kPa during the second part.

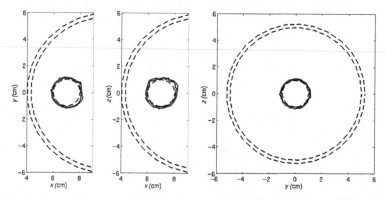

Fig. 11. Feedforward controlled thermal dose contours for 3D simulation. Left: The dose in xy-plane. Middle: The dose in xz-plane. Right: The dose in yz-plane. Contour lines are for 120 and 240 equivalent minutes.

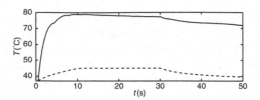

Fig. 12. Maximum temperature trajectories in cancer (solid line) and in healthy subdomains (dotted line) for the 3D feedforward control simulation.

3.5 Feedback control method

The modeling of ultrasound therapy is partly approximate. The main source of error in ultrasound therapy treatment planning is in the acoustic parameters in the Helmholtz equation and in the thermal parameters in the bioheat equation. These errors affect the obtained temperature or thermal dose distribution if the treatment is accomplished by using only the model-based feedforward control. Since the MRI temperature measurements are available during the treatment, it is natural to use this information as a feedback to compensate for the modeling errors.

The feedback controller can be derived by linearizing the nonlinear state equation (5) with respect to feedforward control trajectories for temperature and control input. In this step, the time discretization is also changed. The feedforward control is computed with the time discretization of the order of a second. During ultrasound surgery, the temperature feedback from MRI is obtained in a few second intervals. Due to this mismatch, it is natural to consider the case when feedback is computed with a larger time discretization than the feedforward part. This also reduces the computation task of the feedback controller and filter. Let the step length of the time discretization in feedforward control be h. In feedback control, d steps of the feedforward control are taken at once, giving new step length dh. With these changes the multi-step implicit Euler form of the linearized state equation with the state noise w_k is

$$\Delta T_{k+1} = \widetilde{F} \Delta T_k + \widetilde{B}_k \Delta u_k + w_k, \tag{18}$$

where

$$\widetilde{F} = F^d \tag{19}$$

$$\widetilde{B}_k = h \sum_{t=kd+1}^{kd+d} F^{t-kd-1} G(u_{0,t}), \tag{20}$$

and where $G(u_{0,t})$ is the Jacobian matrix with respect to feedforward input trajectory $u_{0,t}$. The discrete time cost function for the feedback controller can be formulated as

$$\Delta J = \frac{1}{2} \sum_{k=1}^{N_k} \left((\Delta T_k - T_{0,k})^T Q (\Delta T_k - T_{0,k}) + \Delta u_k^T R \Delta u_k \right), \qquad (21)$$

where the error between the feedforward and actual temperature is weighted with matrix Q, and the matrix R weights the correction to the control input. The solution to the control problem can be obtained by computing the associated Riccati difference equation [42].

For the state estimation, the multi-step implicit Euler state equation and the measurement equation are written as

$$\Delta T_{k+1} = \widetilde{F} \Delta T_k + \widetilde{B}_k \Delta u_k + w_k \qquad (22)$$

$$y_k = C \Delta T_k + v_k, \qquad (23)$$

where y_k is the MRI measured temperature, $C \in \mathbb{R}^{P \times N}$ is the linear interpolation matrix and v_k is the measurement noise. When state and measurement noises are independent Gaussian processes with a zero mean, the optimal state estimation can be computed using the Kalman filter. Furthermore, the covariance matrices in this study are assumed to be time independent, so the Kalman filter gain can be computed from the associated Riccati difference equation [42].

The overall feedback control and filtering schemes are applied to the original system via separation principle [42]. In this study, the zero-order hold feedback control is tested using synthetic data. In feedforward control, the acoustic and thermal parameters are adopted from the literature, i.e., they are only approximate values. As the real system is simulated, these parameters are varied. In this case, the original nonlinear state equation (5) with varied parameters and feedback correction can be written as

$$T_{t+1} = A_r T_t + P_r + M_{D,r}(B_r(u_{0,t} + \Delta u_k))^2, \qquad (24)$$

where the feedback correction Δu_k is held constant over the time interval $t \in [k, k+1]$ and subscript r denotes the associated FE matrices which are constructed by using the real parameters.

The state estimate is computed for the same discretization (with step length h) as the state equation with original feedforward control matrices, since errors are considered as unknown disturbances to the system. During the time interval $t \in [k, k+1]$, the state estimate is

$$\widehat{T}_{t+1} = A\widehat{T}_t + P + M_D(B(u_{0,t} + \Delta u_k))^2. \qquad (25)$$

The corrections for the state estimate and the input are updated after every step k from the measurements and the state estimated feedback as

$$y_k = C T_k + v_k \qquad (26)$$

$$\widehat{T}_{k+1} = A\widehat{T}_k + P + M_D \left(B(u_{0,k} + \Delta u_k) \right)^2 + L(y_k - C\widehat{T}_k) \qquad (27)$$

$$\Delta u_{k+1} = -K_{k+1}(\widehat{T}_{k+1} - T_{0,k+1}), \qquad (28)$$

where L is the Kalman gain and K_{k+1} is the LQG feedback gain. The feedback correction is constant during time interval $t \in [k, k+1]$ and piecewise constant during the whole treatment.

3.6 Feedback control simulations

The LQG feedback control algorithm was tested for the 2D example of the feedforward control. The corresponding feedforward control problem is defined in Section 3.4. The time discretization for the feedback controller was set according to the data acquisition time of MRI during in the ultrasound surgery of the breast [27]. The time lag between the MRI measurements was set to 4 s to simulate MRI sequences and temperature measurement in each vertex was taken as a mean value during each 4 s interval. The multi-step implicit Euler equation (18) was adopted by setting $d=8$, since h in feedforward control was 0.5 s. The LQG feedback controller was derived by setting weighting matrices as $Q = W/1000$ for the state weighting and $R=\text{diag}(1000)$ for the input correction weighting. The Kalman filter was derived by setting the state covariance matrix to $\text{diag}(4)$ and the measurement disturbance covariance matrix to identity matrix.

The LQG procedure was tested with simulations, where maximum error in the absorption coefficient was ±50% and ±30% in other acoustic and thermal parameters. New FEM matrices were constructed using these values (matrices with subscript r in Equation (24)). In this study, results from the two worst case simulations are given. In case A, absorption in subdomains is dramatically higher than in feedforward control. In case B, absorption in tissue is lower than in feedforward control. In addition, the other thermal and acoustic parameters are varied in tissue. In both cases, new ultrasound fields were computed with the UWVF.

The acoustic and thermal parameters for the feedback case A are given in Table 4. As compared to Table 3, the acoustic and thermal parameters are changed so that the new parameters result in inhomogeneous errors in temperature trajectories in different subdomains.

The thermal dose contours with and without feedback are shown in Figure 13. This figure indicates that feedback controller decreases undesired thermal dose in healthy regions, while without feedback the healthy breast

Table 4. The acoustic and thermal parameters for the feedback case A.

Domain	α (Nep/m)	c (m/s)	ρ (kg/m^{3}s)	k (W/mK)	C_T (J/kgK)	w_B (kg/m^{3}s)
Ω_2	14	1700	1100	0.60	3650	0.8
Ω_3	7	1500	980	0.70	3600	0.6
Ω_4	8	1400	1000	0.70	3700	2.0

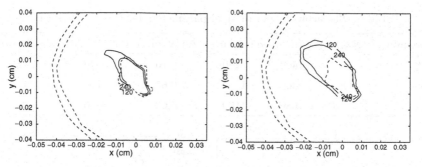

Fig. 13. Thermal dose contours for the feedback case A. Left: Thermal dose with feedback. Right: Thermal dose without feedback.

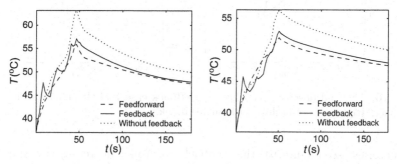

Fig. 14. Temperature trajectories for the feedback case A. Left: Maximum temperature in cancer. Right: Maximum temperature in healthy breast.

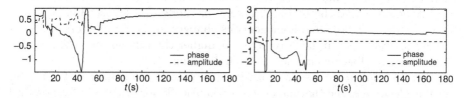

Fig. 15. Phase and amplitude trajectories from the feedback case A for transducer number 4 (left) and 16 (right).

suffers from the undesired damage. The area where thermal dose of 240 equivalent minutes is achieved covers 72% of the cancer region with feedback and 99.4% without feedback. In the healthy breast, the area where thermal dose of 240 equivalent minutes is achieved is 0.7% of the whole region with feedback and 7.9% without feedback.

The maximum temperature trajectories for the feedback case A are shown in Figure 14. The maximum temperature in cancerous and healthy tissue is decreased when the feedback controller is used.

The phase and amplitude trajectories for transducers number 4 and 16 for feedback case A are shown in Figure 15. As compared to original input

Table 5. The acoustic and thermal parameters for the feedback case B.

Domain	α (Nep/m)	c (m/s)	ρ (kg/m³s)	k (W/mK)	C_T (J/kgK)	w_B (kg/m³s)
Ω_2	10	1400	1200	0.70	3570	1.2
Ω_3	4	1300	1100	0.65	3700	1.2
Ω_4	3.5	1680	1100	0.60	3670	2.8

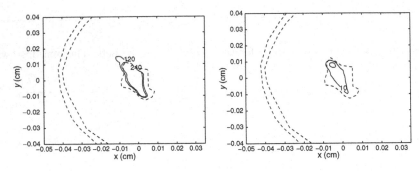

Fig. 16. Thermal dose contours for the feedback case B. Left: Thermal dose with feedback. Right: Thermal dose without feedback.

trajectories (see Figure 9), the feedback controller decreases the amplitude during the first part of the sonication. This is due to the increased absorption in tissue. In addition, the phase is also altered throughout the treatment, since modeling errors are not homogeneously distributed between the subdomains.

The acoustic and thermal parameters for the feedback case B are given in Table 5. Again, there are inhomogeneous changes in the parameters. Furthermore, the absorption in healthy breast is higher than in cancer, which makes the task for feedback controller more challenging.

The thermal dose contours for feedback case B are shown in Figure 16. Without feedback, the thermal dose is dramatically lower than in feedforward control (see Figure 8). With feedback control, the thermal dose distribution is therapeutically relevant in the large part of the cancer, while high thermal dose contours appear in a small part of healthy breast. The area where thermal dose of 240 equivalent minutes is achieved covers 60% of the cancer region with feedback, while without feedback therapeutically relevant dose is not achieved in any part of the target. In healthy breast, the area where thermal dose of 240 equivalent minutes is achieved is 1.8% of the whole region with feedback. In this example, the slight damage to healthy breast was allowed. However, if undesired thermal dose is not allowed in healthy regions, it is possible to increase weighting in the healthy vertices when feedback controller is derived.

Maximum temperature trajectories for feedback case B are shown in Figure 17. The feedback controller increases temperature in cancer effectively. In addition, the temperature in healthy breast does not increase dramatically.

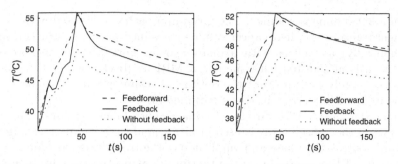

Fig. 17. Temperature trajectories for the feedback case B. Left: Maximum temperature in cancer. Right: Maximum temperature in healthy breast.

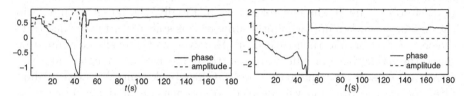

Fig. 18. Phase and amplitude trajectories from the feedback case B for transducer number 4 (left) and 16 (right).

However, during the second part of the sonication, the feedback controller cannot increase the temperature in cancer to compensate modeling errors. This is due to the fact that during this period, transducers were turned effectively off, and the feedback gain is proportional to feedforward control amplitude (for details, see [31]).

The phase and amplitude trajectories for the feedback case B are shown in Figure 18. The feedback controller increases the amplitude to compensate the decreased absorption in tissue. Furthermore, as compared to Figure 9, the phase trajectories are also changed with feedback. This is due to the inhomogeneous modeling errors in subdomains.

4 Conclusions

In this study, alternative control procedures for thermal dose optimization in ultrasound surgery were presented. The presented methods are scanning path optimization methods if prefocused ultrasound fields are used and combined feedforward and feedback control approaches in which the phase and amplitude of the ultrasound transducers are changed as a function of time.

The presented scanning path optimization algorithm is relatively simple. If any kind of treatment planning is made, it would be worth using this kind of approach to find the optimal scanning path. The numerical simulations show that the approach significantly decreases the treatment time, especially when a 3D volume is scanned. The given approach can be used with a single element transducer (where cancer volume is scanned by moving the transducer mechanically) as well as with a phased array. Furthermore, the presented algorithm is also tested with simulated MRI feedback data in [34]. Results from that study indicate that the optimized scanning path is robust even if there are modeling errors in tissue parameters.

The combined feedforward and feedback control method can be applied in cases when the phased array is used in ultrasound surgery treatment. In feedforward control, the phase and amplitude of the transducers are computed as a function of time to optimize the thermal dose. With inequality constraint approximations, it is possible to limit the maximum input amplitude and maximum temperature in tissue. Furthermore, the diffusion and perfusion are taken into account in the control iteration. Finally, the latent accumulating thermal dose is taken into account if sonication is split to parts in which transducers are first on and then turned off. However, as the feedback simulations show, the model based feedforward control is not robust enough if modeling errors are present. For this case, the LQG feedback controller with Kalman filter for state estimation was derived to compensate modeling errors. The main advantage of the proposed feedback controller is that it can change not only the amplitude of the transducers but also the phase. As the results from the simulations show, the phase correction is needed to compensate inhomogeneous modeling errors. The feedback controller increases the robustness of the overall control scheme dramatically.

As the computational task between the proposed approaches are compared, the combined feedforward and feedback approach is computationally much more demanding than the scanning path optimization method. The feedforward control iteration in particular is quite slow due to the large dimensions of the problem. In addition, the associated Riccati matrix equations for feedback controller and Kalman filter have very large dimensions. However, these Riccati equations, as well as the feedforward controller, can be computed off line before actual treatment.

The modeling errors in the model based control of ultrasound surgery can be decreased with pretreatment. In this stage, it is possible to heat tissue with low ultrasound power levels and then measure the thermal response of tissue with MRI. From this data, thermal parameters of tissue can be estimated [23, 46].

References

1. D. Arora, M. Skliar, and R. B. Roemer. Model-predictive control of hyperthermia treatments. *IEEE Transactions on Biomedical Engineering*, 49:629–639, 2002.
2. I. Babuška and J. M. Melenk. The partition of unity method. *International Journal for Numerical Methods in Engineering*, 40:727–758, 1997.

3. J. C. Bamber. Ultrasonic properties of tissue. In F. A. Duck, A. C. Baker, , and H. C. Starrit, editors, *Ultrasound in Medicine*, pages 57–88. Institute of Physics Publishing, 1998. chapter 4.

4. A. B. Bhatia. *Ultrasonic Absorption: An Introduction to the Theory of Sound Absorption and Dispersion in Gases, Liquids and Solids.* Dover, 1967.

5. Y. Y. Botros, J. L. Volakis, P. VanBare, and E. S. Ebbini. A hybrid computational model for ultrasound phased-array heating in the presence of strongly scattering obstacles. *IEEE Transactions on Biomedical Engineering*, 44:1039–1050, 1997.

6. O. Cessenat and B. Després. Application of an ultra weak variational formulation of elliptic PDEs to the two-dimensional Helmholtz problem. *SIAM Journal of Numerical Analysis*, 35:255–299, 1998.

7. A. Chung, F. A. Jolesz, and K. Hynynen. Thermal dosimetry of a focused ultrasound beam *in vivo* by magnetic resonance imaging. *Medical Physics*, 26:2017–2026, 1999.

8. F. P. Curra, P. D. Mourad, V. A. Khokhlova, R. O. Cleveland, , and L. A. Crum. Numerical simulations of heating patterns and tissue temperature response due to high-intensity focused ultrasound. *IEEE Transactions on Ultrasonics, Ferroelectrics, and Frequency Control*, 47:1077–1088, 2000.

9. C. Damianou and K. Hynynen. Focal spacing and near-field heating during pulsed high temperature ultrasound hyperthermia. *Ultrasound in Medicine & Biology*, 19:777–787, 1993.

10. C. Damianou and K. Hynynen. The effect of various physical parameters on the size and shape of necrosed tissue volume during ultrasound surgery. *The Journal of the Acoustical Society of America*, 95:1641–1649, 1994.

11. C. A. Damianou, K. Hynynen, and X. Fan. Evaluation of accuracy of a theoretical model for predicting the necrosed tissue volume during focused ultrasound surgery. *IEEE Transactions on Ultrasonics, Ferroelectrics and Frequency Control*, 42:182–187, 1995.

12. S. K. Das, S. T. Clegg, and T. V. Samulski. Computational techniques for fast hyperthermia optimization. *Medical Physics*, 26:319–328, February 1999.

13. D. R. Daum and K. Hynynen. Thermal dose optimization via temporal switching in ultrasound surgery. *IEEE Transactions on Ultrasonics, Ferroelectrics, and Frequency Control*, 45:208–215, 1998.

14. D. R. Daum and K. Hynynen. Non-invasive surgery using ultrasound. IEEE Potentials, December 1998/January 1999, 1999.

15. F. A. Duck, A. C. Baker, and H. C. Starrit. *Ultrasound in Medicine.* Institute of Physics Publishing, 1998.

16. X. Fan and K. Hynynen. The effect of wave reflection and refraction at soft tissue interfaces during ultrasound hyperthermia treatments. *The Journal of the Acoustical Society of America*, 91:1727–1736, 1992.

17. X. Fan and K. Hynynen. Ultrasound surgery using multiple sonications – treatment time considerations. *Ultrasound in Medicine and Biology*, 22:471–482, 1996.

18. D. Gianfelice, K. Khiat, M. Amara, A. Belblidia, and Y. Boulanger. MR imaging-guided focused US ablation of breast cancer: histopathologic assessment of effectiveness – initial experience. *Radiology*, 227:849–855, 2003.

19. S. A. Goss, R. L. Johnston, and F. Dunn. Compilation of empirical ultrasonic properties of mammalian tissues II. *The Journal of the Acoustical Society of America*, 68:93–108, 1980.

20. L. M. Hocking. *Optimal Control: An Introduction to the theory and applications.* Oxford University Press Inc., 1991.
21. E. Hutchinson, M. Dahleh, and K. Hynynen. The feasibility of MRI feedback control for intracavitary phased array hyperthermia treatments. *International Journal of Hyperthermia*, 14:39–56, 1998.
22. K. Hutchinson and E. B. Hynynen. Intracavitary ultrasound phased arrays for noninvasive prostate surgery. *IEEE Transactions on Ultrasonics, Ferroelectrics and Frequency Control*, 43:1032–1042, 1996.
23. J. Huttunen, T. Huttunen, M. Malinen, and J. P. Kaipio. Determination of heterogeneous thermal parameters using ultrasound induced heating and MR thermal mapping. *Physics in Medicine and Biology*, 51:1102–1032, 2006.
24. T. Huttunen, P. Monk, and J. P. Kaipio. Computational aspects of the ultraweak variational formulation. *Journal of Computational Physics*, 182:27–46, 2002.
25. K. Hynynen. Biophysics and technology of ultrasound hyperthermia. In M. Gautherie, editor, *Methods of External Hyperthermic Heating*, pages 61–115. Springer-Verlag, 1990. Chapter 2.
26. K. Hynynen. Focused ultrasound surgery guided by MRI. *Science & Medicine*, pages 62–71, September/October 1996.
27. K. Hynynen, O. Pomeroy, D. N. Smith, P. E. Huber, N. J. McDannold, J. Kettenbach, J. Baum, S. Singer, and F. A. Jolesz. MR imaging-guided focused ultrasound surgery of fibroadenomas in the breast: A feasibility study. *Radiology*, 219:176–185, 2001.
28. F. Ihlenburg. *Finite Element Analysis of Acoustic Scattering.* Springer-Verlag, 1998.
29. E. Kühnicke. Three-dimensional waves in layered media with nonparallel and curved interfaces: A theoretical approach. *The Journal of the Acoustical Society of America*, 100:709–716, 1996.
30. K. Mahoney, T. Fjield, N. McDannold, G. Clement, and K. Hynynen. Comparison of modeled and observed *in vivo* temperature elevations induced by focused ultrasound: implications for treatment planning. *Physics in Medicine and Biology*, 46:1785–1798, 2001.
31. M. Malinen, S. R. Duncan, T. Huttunen, and J. P. Kaipio. Feedforward and feedback control of the thermal dose in ultrasound surgery. *Applied Numerical Mathematics*, 56:55–79, 2006.
32. M. Malinen, T. Huttunen, and J. P. Kaipio. An optimal control approach for ultrasound induced heating. *International Journal of Control*, 76:1323–1336, 2003.
33. M. Malinen, T. Huttunen, and J. P. Kaipio. Thermal dose optimization method for ultrasound surgery. *Physics in Medicine and Biology*, 48:745–762, 2003.
34. M. Malinen, T. Huttunen, J. P. Kaipio, and K. Hynynen. Scanning path optimization for ultrasound surgery. *Physics in Medicine and Biology*, 50:3473–3490, 2005.
35. D. T. Mast, L. P. Souriau, D.-L. D. Liu, M. Tabei, A. I. Nachman, and R. C. Waag. A k-space method for large scale models of wave propagation in tissue. *IEEE Transactions on Ultrasonics, Ferroelectrics, and Frequency Control*, 48:341–354, 2001.
36. P. M. Meaney, R. L. Clarke, G. R. ter Haar, and I. H. Rivens. A 3-D finite element model for computation of temperature profiles and regions of thermal damage during focused ultrasound surgery exposures. *Ultrasound in Medicine and Biology*, 24:1489–1499, 1998.

37. P. Monk and D. Wang. A least squares method for the Helmholtz equation. *Computer Methods in Applied Mechanics and Engineering*, 175:121–136, 1999.
38. H. H. Pennes. Analysis of tissue and arterial blood temperatures in the resting human forearm. *Journal of Applied Physiology*, 1:93–122, 1948.
39. A. D. Pierce. *Acoustics: An Introduction to its Physical Principles and Applications*. Acoustical Society of America, 1994.
40. S. A. Sapareto and W. C. Dewey. Thermal dose determination in cancer therapy. *International Journal of Radiation Oncology, Biology, Physics*, 10:787–800, June 1984.
41. M. G. Skinner, M. N. Iizuka, M. C. Kolios, and M. D. Sherar. A theoretical comparison of energy sources -microwave, ultrasound and laser- for interstitial thermal therapy. *Physics in Medicine and Biology*, 43:3535–3547, 1998.
42. R .F. Stengel. *Optimal Control and Estimation*. Dover Publications, Inc., 1994.
43. G. ter Haar. Acoustic surgery. Physics Today, pages 29–34, December 2001.
44. G. R. ter Haar. Focused ultrasound surgery. In F. A. Duck, A. C. Baker, and H. C. Starrit, editors, *Ultrasound in Medicine*, pages 177–188. Institute of Physics Publishing, 1998.
45. B. Van Hal. *Automation and performance optimization of the wave based method for interior structural-acoustic problems*. PhD thesis, Katholieke Universitet Leuven, 2004.
46. A. Vanne and K. Hynynen. MRI feedback temperature control for focused ultrasound surgery. *Physics in Medicine and Biology*, 48:31–43, 2003.
47. H. Wan, P. VanBaren, E. S. Ebbini, and C. A. Cain. Ultrasound surgery: Comparison of strategies using phased array systems. *IEEE Transactions on Ultrasonics Ferroelectrics, and Frequency Control*, 43:1085–1098, 1996.
48. G. Wojcik, B. Fornberg, R. Waag, L. Carcione, J. Mould, L. Nikodym, and T. Driscoll. Pseudospectral methods for large-scale bioacoustic models. *IEEE Ultrasonic Symposium Proceedings*, pages 1501–1506, 1997.